Food and Diet in the UK

Series Editor: Cara Acred

Volume 271

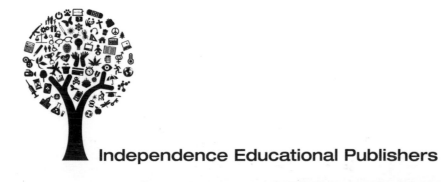

Independence Educational Publishers

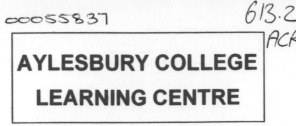

First published by Independence Educational Publishers

The Studio, High Green

Great Shelford

Cambridge CB22 5EG

England

© Independence 2014

British Library Cataloguing in Publication Data

Food and diet in the UK. -- (Issues ; 271)

1. Diet--Great Britain. 2. Food habits--Great Britain.

3. Nutrition--Great Britain. 4. Food industry and trade--

Safety regulations--Great Britain. 5. Food contamination.

I. Series II. Acred, Cara editor.

613.2-dc23

ISBN-13: 9781861686909

Printed in Great Britain
MWL Print Group Ltd

Contents

Chapter 1: How we eat today

How has what we eat changed?	1
Food waste report shows UK families throw away 24 meals a month	2
Walking the breadline	3
Malnutrition	4
Cheese comes from plants and fish fingers are made of chicken	5
Obesity in the UK: analysis and expectations	6
Britain: 'the fat man of Europe'	8
Additives in food	10
The truth about sweeteners	11
There's no debate: lowering salt cuts strokes and heart attacks	12
Thousands of tonnes of saturated fat to be taken out of the nation's diet	13
What is fat?	14
About sugar	16
FactCheck: is sugar really bad for you?	18
'Sugar tax' proposed by campaign group to curb child obesity	20
Why sugar isn't the bad guy	21
Any defence of sugar is pure confection	22

Chapter 2: Make healthier choices

Tips for a healthier diet	23
Understanding food labels	26
Junk food marketing to children campaign	27
Junk foods avoid ad ban by targeting children online	29
Toddlers who eat the same meals as their parents are healthier	30
Healthy eating on a budget	31
FoodSwitch is an addictive app to help find healthier food	32
How do I know if a processed food is high in fat, saturated fat, sugar or salt?	33
The draft School Food Standards	34
Tesco to educate every child about food and where it comes from	35
We would urge the Scottish Government to state clearly that there is no place for Tesco to teach food education in Scottish schools	37
The eatwell plate	39

Key facts	40
Glossary	41
Assignments	42
Index	43
Acknowledgements	44

Introduction

Food and Diet in the UK is Volume 271 in the **ISSUES** series. The aim of the series is to offer current, diverse information about important issues in our world, from a UK perspective.

ABOUT FOOD AND DIET IN THE UK

Concerns surrounding food and diet in the UK are increasing by the day; obesity rates are rising, sugar is the new public enemy, children are unaware that milk comes from cows and many people are simply not financially able to eat a healthy, nutritious, diet. This latest book from the **ISSUES** series explores these controversial topics and considers the steps we can take to achieve a healthier and more nutritionally balanced lifestyle.

OUR SOURCES

Titles in the **ISSUES** series are designed to function as educational resource books, providing a balanced overview of a specific subject.

The information in our books is comprised of facts, articles and opinions from many different sources, including:

⇨ Newspaper reports and opinion pieces

⇨ Website factsheets

⇨ Magazine and journal articles

⇨ Statistics and surveys

⇨ Government reports

⇨ Literature from special interest groups.

A NOTE ON CRITICAL EVALUATION

Because the information reprinted here is from a number of different sources, readers should bear in mind the origin of the text and whether the source is likely to have a particular bias when presenting information (or when conducting their research). It is hoped that, as you read about the many aspects of the issues explored in this book, you will critically evaluate the information presented.

It is important that you decide whether you are being presented with facts or opinions. Does the writer give a biased or unbiased report? If an opinion is being expressed, do you agree with the writer? Is there potential bias to the 'facts' or statistics behind an article?

ASSIGNMENTS

In the back of this book, you will find a selection of assignments designed to help you engage with the articles you have been reading and to explore your own opinions. Some tasks will take longer than others and there is a mixture of design, writing and research-based activities that you can complete alone or in a group.

FURTHER RESEARCH

At the end of each article we have listed its source and a website that you can visit if you would like to conduct your own research. Please remember to critically evaluate any sources that you consult and consider whether the information you are viewing is accurate and unbiased.

Useful weblinks

www.bhf.org.uk

www.bupa.co.uk

www.bwcharity.org.uk

www.theconversation.com

www.eatwell.gov.uk

www.farming.co.uk

www.fifediet.co.uk

lwtww.food.gov.uk

www.foodtank.com

www.ifbb.org.uk

www.nhs.uk

www.noaw.org.uk

www.nutrition.org.uk

www.nutritionist-resource.org.uk

www.oxfam.org.uk

www.patient.co.uk

www.resultsfast.co.uk

www.skillsyouneed.com

www.sugarnutrition.org.uk

How has what we eat changed?

Food and nutrition

Deprived of modern conveniences such as the internal combustion engine and all the labour-saving technology that we take for granted, the lives of the mid-Victorians revolved around manual labour. To fuel their high levels of physical activity they required far more food than we do today; women typically consumed between 3,000 and 3,500 calories per day while men consumed 4,000–5,000 calories, with the navvies, who built the roads, canals and bridges that created the topology of modern Britain, hitting 6,000 or 7,000 calories per day. This compares with an average of around 2,200 today, a figure that we think of as normal but which, at only a relatively small percentage over Basic Metabolic Rate (BMR), is at an historic and unhealthy low.

Given their high calorie intakes you might expect the mid-Victorians to be hugely overweight but early photographs reveal that the mid-Victorians were almost universally

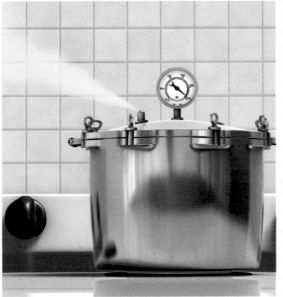

slim and well-muscled. They had the kind of body shapes we can only achieve today by combining regular exercise with dietary restriction – a modern treadmill that most of us cannot stay on for long, as evidenced by the tidal wave of overweight and obesity that is overwhelming modern life.

In mid-Victorian England obesity was virtually unknown except in the numerically small upper-middle and upper classes. The absence of overweight and obesity was a significant factor in their near-freedom from degenerative diseases such as heart disease and cancer, but there were other important factors that contributed to their well-being.

For example, they consumed far less salt, sugar, alcohol and tobacco than we do. They did not use the high temperature cooking methods that today's fast foods demand, and thus were not exposed to the toxins produced when dishes are grilled, deep fried and roasted. They did not consume processed foods (other than the most basic items such as bread, butter, cheese and weak beer), and did not binge on the empty calories that so many of us stuff ourselves with. Perhaps most critically, in the light of the latest recommendations from the cancer specialists, they ate ten or more portions of fruits and vegetables per day. All in all, the mid-Victorian diet contained higher levels of vitamins, minerals and above all phyto-nutrients (nutrients derived from

plants), than occur in today's over-refined, processed and nutrient-poor foods.

The mid-Victorians did not eat a 'super-Mediterranean' diet because they were virtuous, or health-conscious. It's obvious that the health benefits they enjoyed derived from the food choices they made, but food choices depend on food availability and on pricing, both of which were very different from today. Prior to 1900, fruit and vegetables were cheap, as they were mainly grown in allotments or gardens. With the rapid growth of the rail networks and the huge gains in agricultural productivity (the 'agricultural revolution'), large amounts of fresh produce were funnelled into the cities, where the masses now lived. In London 4 lb of freshly picked cherries or a large armful of watercress cost no more than a penny (around £1.50 at today's prices). A poor man's breakfast would have been two chunks of stoneground bread smeared with dripping, accompanied by a large bunch of watercress and often a paper of shrimp or oysters – a meal rich in fibre, protein, vitamins, minerals, omega 3 fatty acids and phyto-nutrients.

They also consumed large amounts of yeast. Bread was whole-meal, generally stone-ground and made daily with yeast; due to their high calorie requirements, mid-Victorians ate five to ten times more bread than we do. The weak beer they drank was unfiltered, and therefore also had a high yeast content. As synthetic fungicides did not emerge until the 1950s almost all other foods were contaminated with yeast, some of which was visible as the spots on apples and pears, or the bloom on plums and grapes.

This high intake of yeast had multiple health benefits. Recent research has proved that yeast enhances innate immune function, leading to improved resistance to infection and a reduced risk of allergy and cancer. Modern food technology has, sadly, removed almost all the yeast from our diets, leaving us vulnerable. For those interested in the details of the mid-Victorian diet, the use of salt as a preservative had faded out by 1850 as improved agricultural productivity made over-winter food hoarding redundant. After that time salt was only used – sparingly – as a flavouring until about 1900, by which time the national diet and the national health had substantially deteriorated. Tobacco was chewed, used in snuff or roll-ups, but overall tobacco consumption was low. This changed in the late 1880s when mass-manufactured cigarettes arrived and began to wreak havoc on public health. At first only the wealthier classes could afford them but as cigarette prices fell an epidemic of tobacco-related cancers and heart disease began to affect the entire population.

⇨ The above information is reprinted with kind permission from IFBB. Please visit www.ifbb.org.uk for further information.

Food waste report shows UK families throw away 24 meals a month

By Rebecca Smithers, consumer affairs correspondent

The average UK family is wasting nearly £60 a month by throwing away almost an entire meal a day, according to a new report that reveals the scale of the ongoing challenge to reduce household food waste.

Britons are chucking out the equivalent of 24 meals a month, adding up to 4.2 million tonnes of food and drink every year that could have been consumed. Almost half of this is going straight from fridges or cupboards into the bin. One-fifth of what households buy ends up as waste, and around 60% of that could have been eaten.

There has been no progress in reducing meat and fish wastage, with Britons still throwing away the equivalent of 86 million chickens every year. The top three foods being thrown away uneaten in British homes are bread, potatoes and milk. The equivalent of 24 million slices of bread, 5.8 million potatoes and 5.9 million glasses of milk are being wasted daily, while even cakes and pastries make it into the top ten most wasted items.

The study by the Government's waste advisory body, the Waste & Resources Action Programme (WRAP), shows that since 2007, avoidable household food waste has been cut by 21% to 4.2 million tonnes, saving consumers almost £13 billion.

WRAP said that such waste should be cut a further 1.7 million tonnes a year by 2025, saving up to £45 billion. Its chief executive, Dr Liz Goodwin, called on retailers, manufacturers, governments and consumers to agree to a 'major combined effort'.

'Consumers are seriously worried about the cost of food and how it has increased over recent years. Yet as WRAP's research shows, we are still wasting millions of tonnes and billions of pounds,' she said.

The main reasons for the waste are shoppers buying more than they need, lack of clarity around storage and labelling and over-estimating portions, WRAP said. The carbon associated with avoidable household food waste is equivalent to taking one in four cars off UK roads.

Last month the UK's largest retailer, Tesco, agreed to reduce its multi-buy items and other promotions after revealing that 35% of its bagged salad is being thrown out. It also found that 40% of apples were wasted, and just under half of bakery items.

Andrew Opie, British Retail Consortium director of food and sustainability, said: 'There's plenty to be pleased about in these figures. Avoidable household food waste has been reduced by 21% since 2007 and the progress is all the more impressive if one accounts for the growth of one million new households within that time. Cutting food waste in the home needs to be one of the UK's biggest environmental priorities.'

He said retailers know they are judged by the value they offer consumers 'which means not only selling food at the right price but also making sure we can make the most of it. A range of approaches, including giving clear storage advice and recipe ideas, offering a wider range of portion sizes, and developing innovative packaging that extends the shelf life of products, has helped to drive significant reductions in the amount of food and drink we throw away.'

• This article was amended on 8 November 2013. The number of chickens thrown away was amended, from 96 million to 86 million. The saving of £13 billion is over a five-year period, not one year, as the article originally stated.

7 November 2013

⇨ The above information is reprinted with kind permission from *The Guardian*. Please visit www.theguardian.com for further information.

Walking the breadline

The scandal of food poverty in 21st-century Britain.

By Niall Cooper and Sarah Dumpleton

The explosion in food poverty and the use of food banks is a national disgrace, and undermines the UK's commitment to ensuring that all its citizens have access to food – one of the most basic of all human rights.

We estimate that over 500,000 people are now reliant on food aid – the use of food banks and receipt of food parcels – and this number is likely to escalate further over the coming months. This is substantially higher than the headline figure of 350,000 supplied by the Trussell Trust, as at least half as many people again are provided with food parcels or other forms of food aid by non-Trussell Trust food banks and other emergency food aid projects.

Some of the increase in the number of people using food banks is caused by unemployment, increasing levels of underemployment, low and falling income, and rising food and fuel prices. The National Minimum Wage and benefits levels need to rise in line with inflation, in order to ensure that families retain the ability to live with dignity and can afford to feed and clothe themselves and stay warm.

More alarmingly, up to half of all people turning to food banks are doing so as a direct result of having benefit payments delayed, reduced, or withdrawn altogether. Figures gathered by the Trussell Trust show that changes to the benefit system are the most common reasons for people using food banks; these include changes to crisis loan eligibility rules, delays in payments, Jobseeker's Allowance sanctions and sickness benefit reassessments.

There is clear evidence that the benefit sanctions regime has gone too far, and is leading to destitution, hardship and hunger on a large scale.

There is a real risk that the benefit cuts and the introduction of Universal Credit (which will require Internet access and make payments less frequently) will lead to even larger numbers being forced to turn to food banks. Food banks may not have the capacity to cope with the increased level of demand.

The growth in food aid demonstrates that the social safety net is failing in its basic duty to ensure that families have access to sufficient income to feed themselves adequately. The exponential rise in the creation of food banks reflects a growing problem and only delivers mitigation. Food banks provide a vital emergency service to the people they support but they do not address the underlying structural causes for the growth of food poverty.

Food banks should not replace the 'normal' safety net provided by the state in the form of the welfare state. Even in developing countries, food aid is increasingly seen only as an emergency stop-gap measure. International practice would now indicate a preference for cash payments over food handouts, not least because they distort local markets and are not part of a long-term development or anti-poverty strategy.

It is unacceptable that whilst thousands are being forced to turn to food banks and millions are unable to meet the rising cost of living as a result of the Government's austerity programme, wealthy individuals and corporations continue to dodge their obligation to pay their fair share of taxes.

Recommendations

1. The House of Commons Work and Pensions Select Committee conducts an urgent inquiry into the relationship between benefit delay, error or sanctions, welfare reform changes, and the growth of food poverty.

2. The Department for Work and Pensions publishes data on a regular basis on the number and type of household who are deprived of their benefits by reason of benefit delay, error or sanctions; the numbers leaving and returning to benefits after a short period of time, and the number of referrals from Jobcentre staff to local food banks.

3. The Department for Work and Pensions commission independent monitoring of the roll-out of Universal Credit, to ensure that there is no unintentional increase in food poverty.

4. All referrals to food banks/ emergency food aid provision, made by government agencies, be recorded and monitored in order to establish more accurate numbers on people experiencing food poverty in the UK.

5. HM Treasury make tackling tax dodging an urgent priority, including promoting robust and coordinated international action at the forthcoming G8 meeting in Northern Ireland in June – to reduce the need for future cuts in benefits, and restore the principle that benefits should at least rise in line with inflation.

May 2013

Malnutrition

Malnutrition essentially means 'poor nutrition' – when the human body contains an insufficient, excessive or imbalanced consumption of nutrients.

The two types of malnutrition are:

Undernutrition (subnutrition) – When a person's diet is lacking in nutrients and does not provide them with an adequate amount of calories, sustenance and protein for maintenance and growth. Undernutrition can also occur if the body cannot efficiently use food as a result of an illness.

Overnutrition – When a person's diet is getting far too many nutrients for the body to cope with. Usually a result of people choosing to eat more food than they need, but in rare cases can be caused by excessive supplement intake.

Malnutrition can affect people of all ages, gender and health, although it tends to be more common in developing countries where there are shortages of food. In industrialised countries however, more and more people are being diagnosed with the condition, with factors such as diet, alcoholism, mental health problems and digestive disorders cited as common causes.

According to the World Health Organization (WHO), malnutrition is the most dangerous single threat to global public health – especially as it can impact significantly on both physical and emotional well-being.

Causes of malnutrition

Poor diet

As explained above, the most common causes of malnutrition are diet-related – getting too much, or not enough food. In less-developed countries many people will develop undernutrition as a result of food shortages and famine.

In more wealthy and industrialised nations such as the UK, food is more accessible but a vast majority of it is fatty, sugary and devoid of any nutritional value. When our diets become too heavily laden with these types of foods our health suffers and we can start to develop symptoms of malnutrition that reflect overnutrition.

Illness and medical conditions

Illnesses and health problems can also cause malnutrition, especially as they can impact eating habits. For example, if an illness leaves a patient with symptoms of dysphagia (difficulty swallowing), they may not be able to consume enough of the foods that they need for healthy nutrition.

Digestive disorders and stomach conditions are further causes of malnutrition. Crohn's disease for example disrupts the body's ability to digest food and absorb vital nutrients, meaning the patient's health can suffer. On the other hand, people who suffer from digestive complaints such as IBS might avoid eating certain foods, which means they could be missing out on vital nutrition.

Mental health problems

People suffering from mental health problems are more likely to have poor nutrition as they can find it difficult to look after themselves properly, especially if they struggle to communicate their needs to carers. Research conducted by Alzheimer's Disease International (ADI) revealed that half of people with dementia and Alzheimer's will end up showing signs of malnutrition.

Depression can also impact our diets and how we look after ourselves, while people suffering from more acute psychological disorders such as anorexia nervosa and bulimia will severely limit the amount of food they consume and how many nutrients can be absorbed through the digestive process.

Physical factors

A whole host of physical factors can contribute to poor nutrition. If a person has a disability or impairment, they may find it difficult to go shopping and even cook. Poor dental hygiene, such as badly fitting dentures or painful gums can also prevent people from eating properly and getting the right amount of nutrients. A lost sense of smell or taste can put people off eating altogether.

Social factors

The environment can significantly impact diet, and people surviving on low incomes and/or in poverty are more likely to develop symptoms of malnutrition. Although malnutrition due to inadequate food intake in the UK is rare, there are still circumstances where neglect and poverty can lead to undernutrition, particularly in children. Living alone and being socially isolated may also affect a person's eating habits, while those suffering from alcohol or drug dependencies are likely to have little appetite.

Taking too many nutritional supplements

While overnutrition is commonly associated with overeating, it can also stem from taking too many nutritional supplements. Many people take vitamins and supplements as part of a healthy diet and lifestyle, but in rare cases excessive consumption can lead to vitamin and iron poisoning. Synthetic nutritional supplements should be taken with caution and you should always consult a medical professional before taking supplements as a means of correcting a severe deficiency.

Effects of malnutrition

As well as the various symptoms of malnutrition, the condition can also lead to complex health conditions that can greatly affect overall well-being.

Effects of undernutrition

For those who are undereating, usually the effects of malnutrition will only occur if a calorie and nutrient deficiency continues for a period of time.

Some of the most common side effects of undernutrition include: respiratory failure, higher risk of hypothermia and pneumonia, weaker immune system thus increased risk of catching an infection and longer recovery time, poor wound healing, fertility problems, organ failure, urinary infections, development of health conditions such as edema, anaemia and jaundice, total starvation could be fatal if no calories have been consumed for a long period of time.

There can also be severe consequences that result from specific micronutrient deficiencies in someone's diet, such as anaemia (iron deficiency) or scurvy (vitamin c deficiency).

Effects of overnutrition

For those suffering from overnutrition, effects on physical and emotional health will be very similar to those caused by undernutrition.

However, debilitating obesity-related illnesses such as type 2 diabetes, high blood pressure and gallstones will exacerbate these.

⇨ The above information is reprinted with kind permission from Nutritionist Resource.

Cheese comes from plants and fish fingers are made of chicken

Research conducted by the British Nutrition Foundation (BNF) among over 27,500 children across the UK, shows that nearly a third (29 per cent) of primary school children think that cheese comes from plants, one in ten secondary school children believe that tomatoes grow under the ground, and nearly one in five (18 per cent) primary school children say that fish fingers come from chicken.

The survey, the largest of its kind, was conducted as part of the BNF's Healthy Eating Week, launched today by HRH The Princess Royal. More than 3,000 schools are participating in the week during which over 1.2 million children will be learning valuable lessons about healthy eating, cooking and where foods come from.

Roy Ballam, Education Programme Manager at the British Nutrition Foundation, said: 'Schools throughout the UK require a national framework and guidance for food and nutrition education to support the learning needs of children and young people, especially at a time when levels of childhood obesity are soaring. Through Healthy Eating Week, we hope to start the process of re-engaging children with the origins of food, nutrition and cooking, so that they grow up with a fuller understanding of how food reaches them and what a healthy diet and lifestyle consists of. The fact that so many schools in England, Northern Ireland, Scotland and Wales have registered to participate in the week demonstrates their understanding of how important healthy eating is and their commitment to giving children a solid grounding from which to create healthy lives for themselves.'

Further findings of the BNF study reveal that an encouraging number of the youngest primary school children recognise the eatwell plate – 64 per cent of 5–8-year-olds identified it correctly from four different images. However, when presented with four pie charts and asked which best represented the eatwell plate, less than half (45 per cent) of 8–11-year-olds answered correctly.

Over three quarters (77 per cent) of primary school children and nearly nine out of every ten (88 per cent) secondary school pupils know that people should consume five or more portions of fruit and vegetables each day. However, 67 per cent of primary school children and 81 per cent of secondary school pupils reported eating four or less portions of fruit and vegetables daily, while two in every five children at secondary school don't think that frozen fruit and vegetables count towards their five a day.

The research also shows that an alarming number of children do not eat breakfast each morning, which increases with the age of the children. On the day of the survey, eight per cent of primary school children said they hadn't eaten breakfast that morning; this increased to nearly a quarter (24 per cent) in 11–14-year-olds, and then to over a third (32 per cent) of 14–16-year-olds. When quizzed on the more general point as to whether they have breakfast each morning, six per cent of primary school children, 19 per cent of 11–14-year-olds and a quarter of 14–16-year-olds reported not eating breakfast every day.

Scientific evidence confirms that consumption of fish, in particular oily fish, is beneficial to health. National recommendations are that children and adults should consume at least two portions of fish each week. However, in the BNF survey 16 per cent of children of primary school age and one in five children of secondary school age said they never eat fish. Averaged across all age groups, from five- to 16-year-olds, only 17 per cent of children in the UK said they eat fish twice a week.

The BNF research also looks at reported home cooking behaviour and shows that 17 per cent of primary school children and 19 per cent of secondary school children cook at home either every day or once a week. However, nine per cent of children at primary school and 11 per cent of children at secondary school never cook at home. Encouragingly, 84 per cent of primary school children and nearly three quarters (73 per cent) of secondary school children would like to cook more and an average of 85 per cent of children across all age groups say that they enjoy cooking.

Ballam concluded: 'Through this survey one in five (21 per cent) primary school children and 18 per cent of secondary school pupils told us that they have never visited a farm. This may go part way to explaining why over a third (34 per cent) of 5–8-year-olds and 17 per cent of 8–11-year-olds believe that pasta comes from animals.'

⇨ The above information is reprinted with kind permission from The British Nutrition Foundation 2013. Please visit www.nutrition.org.uk for further information.

Obesity in the UK: analysis and expectations

Scale of obesity in the UK – an overview

The Foresight report (2007) concluded that half the UK population could be obese by 2050 at a cost of £50 billion per year. However, upward trends in obesity levels suggest these conclusions could be optimistic and could be exceeded by 2050.

The current state of the UK is set out separately, but it is useful to provide a brief overview of the situation in order to establish the context within which existing policies and initiatives can be assessed.

Research by the Health & Social Care Information Centre has demonstrated sharp and substantial increases in obesity levels amongst adults and children between 1993 and 2011.[1] This has not only included Body Mass Indices (BMI) within the overweight and obese ranges, but also an increasing number of individuals with raised waist circumferences. These finding should be taken very seriously in any event given their source, but are backed by separate studies on adult obesity levels by the University of Glasgow[2] (that has demonstrated evidence of people getting fatter later in life), and levels of childhood obesity by Leeds Metropolitan University.[3]

It should, however, be noted that the most recent figures published by the Health & Social Care Information Centre has shown a fall in the number of obese and overweight children in their final year of primary school in England for the first time in six years[4] – although this is counterbalanced by the facts that childhood obesity levels remain worryingly high and that any levelling off in obesity rates tends to be amongst the children of more affluent families. High levels of obesity amongst children in deprived areas remain.

Despite the most recent statistics of levels of English childhood obesity, the sum of these studies is a disturbing picture.

The effectiveness of government policy

'We are failing too many of our children, women and young people on a grand scale. Health inequality, arising from social and economic inequalities, are socially unjust, unnecessary and unavoidable.'[5] (Professor Sir Michael Marmot)

Government policy on the subjects of weight management and obesity is analysed and assessed at length later in this article. However, it is worth briefly summarising what initiatives, projects and policies are currently in place, and to make some initial comments regarding their effectiveness that will be expanded upon throughout this article.

The public and business

Two of the flagship government initiatives in this area are the Change4Life programme and the Public Health Responsibility Deal. The former was established in light of the 2007 Foresight report, from which the government of the day clearly established that an obesity problem existed in the UK. Change4Life is intended to provide the public with advice on healthy diets and physical activity.

The Responsibility Deal was established to encourage businesses, including food and drink manufacturers and retailers, to do their part in reducing obesity levels by making it easier for individuals and families to make healthy choices. The Responsibility Deal has a collection of pledges that businesses are encouraged to commit to. This includes reducing the likes of salt and fat that can be harmful in products, encouraging people to reach their 'five-a-day' of fruit and vegetables and reduce their saturated fat intake, putting calorie information on menus and products, and helping individuals to reduce their calorie consumption.

Schools

Successive governments have introduced guidance and requirements for schools on food standards relating to school meals, although not including packed lunches brought from home. These include guidance on what school meals are to include and what schools are not allowed to provide to pupils.

There have also been a range of additions to pupils' curriculums to help promote knowledge of healthy eating and participation in physical activity. This has included the School Food Plan and the introduction of cookery/food technology lessons that are intended to provide pupils with knowledge of how to cook, and of healthy eating.

An announcement by the Department for Education (DfE) in September 2013 also committed schools to a new national curriculum for physical education. All schools are required to deliver physical education to pupils in all four key stages of education. The DfE announcement of September 2013 introduced a new focus on competitive sport and increased physical activity. Additional funding of £150 million was also announced to improve the provision of physical education and sport in primary schools.

General practitioners

General practitioners (GPs) have been subject to the Quality Outcomes Framework (QOF), a voluntary incentive-based initiative that measures and financially rewards GPs and their surgeries for delivery on a wide range of indicators.

This has included indicators on obesity and on physical activity. However, the process for determining the indicators is a complex one and QOF is expected to undergo significant change in the coming months.

1   Health & Social Care Information Centre, Statistics on obesity, physical activity and diet (England), 2013

2   Vlassopoulos, A., Combet, E. & Lean, E.J., 'Changing distributions of body size and adiposity with age', International Journal of Obesity, 2013

3   Griffiths, C., Gately, P., Marchant, P.R., Cooke, C.B., 'A five year longitudinal study investigating the prevalence of childhood obesity', Journal of Public Health, November 2013

4   'Obesity falls in English schools', BBC News (http://www.bbc.co.uk/news/health-25331997), 12 December 2013

5   Collins, N., 'Britain faces 'public health time bomb'', Daily Telegraph, 30 October 2013

The indicator on obesity has to date only required GPs to register their obese patients. There is no requirement for them to take action or to engage their patients in discussions about weight management during the course of medical appointments, during which the patient is unlikely to present themselves with concerns about their weight but will instead present issues that are clearly weight related.

Healthy living rather than healthy eating

It would be wrong to roundly criticise government policy. Initiatives such as Change4Life are extremely important in helping to educate the public and promote better choices. Similarly the Responsibility Deal reflects the self-evident fact that business and the food and drink industry must be on-side if issues of weight and obesity are to be effectively addressed.

There are, however, significant gaps that must be addressed.

An individual's intake of salt, trans fats and sugar remains enormously important. Issues such as proper hydration are also largely being overlooked in favour of healthy eating. A study conducted in 2012 by researchers at the University of North Carolina demonstrated a 2%–2.5% average weight loss amongst adults who swapped calorific beverages for non-calorific ones (e.g. water) over a six-month period[6] as a weight loss strategy. A separate UK study measuring the water consumption of children over a 14-day period has also concluded that children display poor hydration habits and are not getting enough water in the morning.[7] This conclusion, while concerning, is not limited to the UK. Similar studies have reached the same conclusions about French school children.[8]

6   Tate, D.F., Turner-McGrievy, G., Lyons, E., Stevens, J., Erikson, K., Polzien, K., Diamond, M., Wang, X., Popkin, B., 'Replacing calorific beverages with water or diet beverages for weight loss in adults', 2012 (randomised clinical trial)

7   Derbyshire, E.J., 'An intervention to improve cognition and hydration in UK school children using bottled water', 2012

8   Bonnet, F. et al., 'French children start their day with a hydration deficit', 2012

While these studies provide only a snapshot, they are indicative of a wider body of evidence demonstrating the effectiveness of proper hydration as part of a broader approach to healthy living rather than an emphasis on healthy eating specifically. This is best demonstrated by the so-called 'eatwell plate'[9] that identifies the different proportions of food to achieve a balanced diet. Minimal guidance is provided as to what one should drink, when poor drinking habits can undermine any amount of healthy eating.

In spite of the efforts of Change4Life and also new initiatives for physical education in schools, the important of physical activity also tends to take a backseat to healthy eating.

Prevention rather than cure

It also remains the case that many governmental interventions, policies and initiatives are focused on the promotion of healthy eating/living for individuals who, while potentially having some weight management issues, are not obese – and indeed may never be.

Comparatively little in the way of support and guidance exists for individuals who find themselves in the position of being obese or even morbidly obese. There are similarly significant deficiencies in GP knowledge of weight management as an issue. Questions should also be asked as to the level of GP knowledge

9   NHS choices website (http://www.nhs.uk/Livewell/Goodfood/Pages/eatwell-plate.aspx)

of the support services for the obese and overweight that will exist, including those in their local communities.

Summary

Weight management and obesity represent significant public health issues for the UK, and it is entirely reasonable to conclude that the determinations of the 2007 Foresight report (i.e. that half the population might be obese by 2050 at an annual cost of nearly £50 billion), while shocking at the time, may now underestimate the scale of the problem.

Clear evidence exists of a substantial proportion of children being overweight or obese, and while recent figures have suggested the situation may be improving, should still cause concern. This, as noted above, is particularly troubling in light of evidence that also suggests people are getting fatter in later life. Should children already be in the position of being overweight or obese by the time they reach their adulthood and later years, it is likely that these problems will not only continue but will be exacerbated.

January 2014

⇨   The above information is reprinted with kind permission from National Obesity Awareness Week. Please visit www.noaw.org.uk for further information.

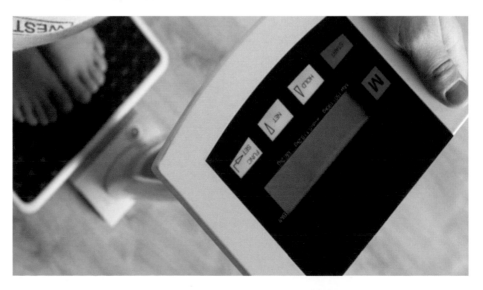

Britain: 'the fat man of Europe'

One in four British adults is obese, according to the UN Food and Agriculture Organisation, prompting fears that the UK has become the 'fat man of Europe'.

The UK has the highest level of obesity in Western Europe, ahead of countries such as France, Germany, Spain and Sweden, the 2013 report says.

Obesity levels in the UK have more than trebled in the last 30 years and, on current estimates, more than half the population could be obese by 2050.

The cause of the rapid rise in obesity has been blamed on our modern lifestyles, including the prevalence of the car, TVs, computers, desk-bound jobs and high-calorie food.

'The UK is the "fat man" of Europe,' writes Professor Terence Stephenson in *Measuring Up*, a 2013 report on the nation's obesity crisis by the Academy of Medical Royal Colleges (AoMRC).

'It is no exaggeration to say that it is the biggest public health crisis facing the UK today,' he says.

The consequences of obesity on our health include diabetes, heart disease and cancer, and people dying needlessly from avoidable diseases.

Britain has become an 'obese society' where being overweight is 'normal'. It is a trend three decades in the making which, according to experts, will take several more to reverse.

Obesity epidemic in numbers

A person is considered overweight if they have a body mass index (BMI) between 25 and 29, and obese with a BMI of 30 and above.

In England, 24.8% of adults are obese and 61.7% are either overweight or obese, according to the Health and Social Care Information Centre.

Today's obesity levels are more than three times what they were in 1980, when only 6% of men and 8% of women were obese.

Most people who become obese put on weight gradually between the ages of 20 and 40, but there is some suggestion that the path is set in early childhood.

'Overweight children are more likely to become overweight adults,' says Susan Jebb, professor of diet and population health at the University of Oxford.

The risk of becoming obese is thought to start at an early age and obesity in a parent increases the risk of childhood obesity by 10%. In 2011, around three in ten boys and girls (aged two to 15) were either overweight or obese and around 16% were obese. The number of children aged 13 to 19 having weight loss surgery has risen from one a year in 2000 to 31 in 2009.

The North East had the highest obesity rates in England at 13.5% during 2011/12 while the South West reported the lowest levels at 10.4%. Tamworth in Staffordshire, where nearly 31% of people were obese, had the unenviable title of being dubbed Britain's fattest town by the media.

'Obesity is closely linked to deprivation levels,' says Dr Alison Tedstone, Director of Diet and Obesity at Public Health England. 'The association is especially strong with children. Children in poor communities are far more likely to be obese.'

Income, social deprivation and ethnicity have an important impact on the likelihood of becoming obese. For example, women and children in lower socioeconomic groups are more likely to be obese than those who are wealthier.

What caused the obesity crisis?

Recent research has challenged the idea that obesity is simply the result of the individual 'eating too much and doing too little'.

Rising obesity is not the result of a national collapse in willpower. Studies have shown the environment has a major influence on the decisions people make about their lifestyle. Known as 'obesogenic environments', these are places, often urban, that encourage unhealthy eating and inactivity.

The car, TV, computers, desk jobs, high-calorie food and clever food marketing have all contributed to encourage inactivity and overeating.

'Obesity is a consequence of the abundance and convenience of modern life as well as the human body's propensity to store fat,' says Professor Jebb.

Research has shown that we have a natural tendency to store fat – it's a survival mechanism that helped early humans survive famine and food shortages. 'The situation in which food is readily available for most people has arrived in a blink of an eye in evolutionary terms,' says Professor Jebb.

Adults spend about six hours a day engaged in sedentary pursuits (watching TV and other screen time, reading and other low-energy activities). On average, men and women spend 2.8 hours watching television per weekday and this rises to about three hours on weekends.

The average distance a person walked for transport purposes has fallen from 255 miles in 1976 to 192 miles in 2003, while car use increased by more than 10%. Although people are travelling further to get to work, one in five journeys of less than one mile are made by car.

'Your likelihood of being active is shaped by the environment you live in,' says Professor Jebb. 'For example, you're more likely to ride a bike if there are safe and convenient cycle lanes.'

In 2008, only 39% of men and 29% of women aged 16 and over met the Government's recommendations for physical activity of 150 minutes a week. Among children aged two to 15, more boys (32%) than girls (24%) met the recommendation to do an hour of activity every day.

Leisure time is increasingly spent indoors whereas the incentives for outdoor play have fallen due to safety concerns and a lack of access to green spaces and sports facilities.

Longer working hours and more desk-bound jobs over the past decades have resulted in limiting opportunities for other forms of activity during the working day.

Breastfeeding, healthy weaning practices and the mother's own diet have all been linked to reduced obesity later in life although why this is the case has yet to be fully explained.

Obesity's health consequences

Being overweight or obese increases the risk of a many serious illnesses, such as type 2 diabetes, high blood pressure, heart disease, stroke, as well as cancer.

'People are dying needlessly from avoidable diseases,' wrote Professor Stephenson in the AoMRC's *Measuring Up* report.

Compared with a healthy weight man, an obese man is:

⇨ five times more likely to develop type 2 diabetes

⇨ three times more likely to develop cancer of the colon

⇨ more than two and a half times more likely to develop high blood pressure – a major risk factor for stroke and heart disease.

An obese woman, compared with a healthy weight woman, is:

⇨ almost 13 times more likely to develop type 2 diabetes

⇨ more than four times more likely to develop high blood pressure

⇨ more than three times more likely to have a heart attack.

People from some ethnic groups, including south Asians, who are more likely to be overweight and obese, also have a higher risk of type 2 diabetes and other weight-related illnesses.

A BMI of 30 to 35 has been found to reduce life expectancy by an average of three years, while a BMI of over 40 reduced longevity by eight to ten years, which is equivalent to a lifetime of smoking.

'As a society, we are gradually realising that obesity poses just as serious a health threat as smoking,' says Dr Tedstone.

Obesity has been blamed for about 30,000 deaths a year in the UK, 9,000 of those taking place before retirement age.

Alongside disease, obesity can affect peoples' ability to get and hold down work, their self-esteem and their well-being and mental health.

What are we doing about it?

Reversing the obesity trend will require society as a whole to think differently. For government and businesses, it means creating an environment that encourages healthier eating and physical activity. For individuals and families, it means eating less and moving more.

It will require a major shift in thinking, not just by government, but by individuals, families, business and society as a whole.

Currently, no country in the world has a comprehensive, long-term strategy to deal with the challenges posed by obesity.

The only country to have successfully reversed its obesity problem was Cuba, although it was the unexpected consequence of an economic downturn in the early 1990s. This caused severe food and fuel shortages, which resulted in an average weight loss per citizen of 5.5 kg over the course of the five-year economic crisis. During this time there was a significant drop in prevalence of, and deaths due to, cardiovascular diseases, type 2 diabetes and cancers.

A study based on the Cuban experience concludes that national initiatives encouraging people to eat less and exercise more could be effective at tackling obesity levels.

The UK Government has recognised that past efforts have not succeeded in turning the tide and that a new approach is required.

In 2011, it published *Healthy Lives, Healthy People*, a policy document setting out its vision for how society as a whole can work together to turn the tide on obesity by 2020. Some of the Government's measures to help people make healthier choices include:

⇨ giving people advice on healthier food choices and physical activity through the Change4Life programme

⇨ improving labelling on food and drink to help people make healthy choices

⇨ encouraging businesses on the high street to include calorie information on their menus so people can make healthy choices

⇨ giving people guidance on how much physical activity they should be doing.

The Government has also asked businesses to play their part in helping everyone – from staff to customers – make healthier choices through its Responsibility Deal pledges.

Food manufacturers, retailers and the hospitality sector have committed to cutting down on the amount of fat, sugar and salt in popular food products, encouraging people to eat more fruit and vegetables, reducing portion sizes and putting calorie information on menus.

Each of us is ultimately responsible for our own health. We should be free to make choices about diet and physical activity for ourselves and for our families.

'However, supermarkets and food manufacturers are already making choices for us by deciding how much fat and sugar to put in their products and what items to stock and promote,' says Professor Jebb.

'Government can play a positive role in working with the private sector to help people make healthier choices to prevent weight gain.'

Given all the external causes of the obesity epidemic, for the individual, it boils down to the simple message: to lose weight, you need to eat less and move more.

'People don't choose to be obese,' says Professor Jebb. 'It just happens for a number of reasons. We should stop blaming people for being fat and instead support them in controlling their weight.

'We've all got the potential to be fat. In the environment we live in, it's easy to overeat and be less active. Some people need to work harder than others at keeping weight gain in check.'

6 November 2013

⇨ The above information is reprinted with kind permission from NHS Choices. Please visit www.nhs.uk for further information.

Additives in food

Additives must be assessed for safety before they can be used in food. We also ensure that the science on additives is strictly reviewed, the law strictly enforced, and action is taken where problems are found. We investigate any information that casts reasonable doubt on the safety of an additive.

European Union (EU) legislation requires most additives used in foods to be labelled clearly in the list of ingredients, with their function, followed by either their name or E number. An E number means that it has passed safety tests and has been approved for use here and in the rest of the EU.

What are the different types of additives?

Food additives are grouped by what they do. The additives that you are most likely to come across on food labels are:

⇨ antioxidants (stop food becoming rancid or changing colour by reducing the chance of fats combining with oxygen)

⇨ colours

⇨ emulsifiers, stabilisers, gelling agents and thickeners (help to mix or thicken ingredients)

⇨ flavour enhancers (used to bring out the flavour of foods)

⇨ preservatives (used to keep food safer for longer)

⇨ sweeteners (intense sweeteners are many times sweeter than sugar whereas bulk sweeteners have a similar sweetness to sugar).

Food additives and children's behaviour

Research undertaken by Southampton University suggests that eating or drinking some artificial food colours could be linked to a negative effect on children's behaviour. In light of these findings, the Food Standards Agency (FSA) has revised its advice to consumers.

In short, the advice states: if a child shows signs of hyperactivity or Attention Deficit Hyperactivity Disorder (ADHD), eliminating the colours considered in the Southampton study from their diet might have some beneficial effects on their behaviour. Qualitative research was commissioned to gauge parents' response to the revised advice. More specifically, research was intended to examine parents' understanding of food additives, including:

⇨ the effects these can have on behaviour

⇨ their awareness of Southampton University's study

⇨ their grasp of the implications of this work

⇨ to explore parents' understanding of the FSA's updated advice, including:

• perceptions on the target audience

• thoughts on relevance/importance of the advice

• views on the practical implications of the advice

• their preferences for how the advice should be communicated.

High caffeine energy drinks and other foods containing caffeine

Energy drinks are generally drinks with high caffeine levels that are claimed by the manufacturers to give the consumer more 'energy' than a typical soft drink.

Energy drinks can contain high levels of caffeine, usually about 80 milligrams (mg) of caffeine in a small 250 ml can – the same as three cans of cola or a mug of instant coffee. As well as caffeine, they may contain other ingredients, such as glucuronolactone and taurine, and sometimes vitamins and minerals or herbal substances. Some of the smaller 'shot style' products can contain anywhere from 80 mg to as much as 175 mg of caffeine in a 60 ml bottle.

Children, or other people sensitive to caffeine, should only consume caffeine in moderation. Pregnant women are advised not to have more than 200 mg of caffeine a day, roughly two mugs of instant coffee. Drinks like espresso and lattes, which are made from ground coffee, typically contain higher levels of caffeine per mug.

Statutory labelling

Drinks containing more than 150 mg of caffeine per litre (mg/l) must be labelled with the term 'high caffeine content' in the same field of vision as the name of the food, which must be accompanied by an indication of the amount of caffeine per 100 ml in the product. No other labelling is currently required by law and this labelling does not apply to drinks such as tea and coffee.

New labelling legislation (The Food Information Regulation (EU) 1169/2011), which will apply from 13 December 2014, will require additional caffeine labelling for high caffeine drinks and foods where caffeine is added for a physiological effect. The requirements are listed on the Food Standards Agency website.

⇨ The above information is reprinted with kind permission from the Food Standards Agency. Please visit www.food.gov.uk for further information.

The truth about sweeteners

Artificial sweeteners: chemical cocktails or a potent weapon in the fight against tooth decay, diabetes and obesity?

Whatever your opinion, there's no avoiding them. They are found in thousands of products, from drinks, desserts and ready meals, to cakes, chewing gum and toothpaste.

Fears about their potential toxic effects have been around ever since the first sweetener, saccharin – once known as 'the poor man's sugar' – was discovered in 1879.

Cancer, strokes, seizures, low birthweight, high blood pressure, vomiting, dizziness – all have been cited as risks from consuming sweeteners.

But none of these claims have stuck, and demand for sweeteners continues unabated as consumers try to cut their sugar intake while still satisfying their sweet tooth.

The UK sweetener sector is valued at £60 million, and more than a quarter of British households buy artificial sweeteners.

Sweeteners are low-calorie or calorie-free chemical substances that are used instead of sugar to sweeten foods and drinks.

Find out what the evidence says on the safety of some of the most common sweeteners approved for use in the UK:

⇨ acesulfame K

⇨ aspartame

⇨ saccharin

⇨ sorbitol

⇨ sucralose

⇨ steviol glycosides (stevia plant extracts)

⇨ xylitol.

All sweeteners in the EU will have undergone a rigorous safety assessment by the European Food Safety Authority (EFSA) or its predecessor, the Scientific Committee on Food (SCF), before they can be used in food and drink.

Moreover, Cancer Research UK and the US National Cancer Institute have said there is no evidence that sweeteners are associated with cancer risk in humans.

'Studies on artificial sweeteners have found that they do not increase the risk of cancer,' states Cancer Research UK.

'Large studies looking at people have now provided strong evidence that artificial sweeteners are safe for humans.'

As part of the evaluation process, the EFSA sets an acceptable daily intake (ADI), which is the maximum amount considered safe to consume each day over the course of your lifetime.

You don't need to keep track of how much sweetener you consume each day, as our eating habits are factored in when specifying where sweeteners can be used.

Are sweeteners healthy?

Safe, yes, but are they healthy? Food manufacturers claim sweeteners help prevent tooth decay, control blood sugar levels and reduce our calorie intake.

EFSA has approved the health claims made about xylitol, sorbitol and sucralose, among others, in relation to oral health and controlling blood sugar levels.

Polyols are a type of sugar-free carbohydrate generally manufactured from sugars and starches. The polyols licensed in the EU are:

⇨ Xylitol E967

⇨ Sorbitol E420

⇨ Mannitol (E421)

⇨ Isomalt (E953)

⇨ Maltitol (E965)

⇨ Lactitol (E966)

⇨ Erythritol (E968).

Polyols are banned from soft drinks in the EU because of their laxative effect.

Dietitian Emma Carder states: 'Research into sweeteners shows they are perfectly safe to eat or drink on a daily basis as part of a healthy diet.'

She also says they are a really useful alternative for people with diabetes who need to watch their blood sugar levels while still enjoying their favourite foods.

'Like sugar, sweeteners provide a sweet taste to foods and drinks, but what sets them apart is that, after consumption, sweeteners don't increase blood sugar levels,' she says.

It has been suggested that the use of artificial sweeteners may have a stimulating effect on appetite and, therefore, may play a role in weight gain and obesity. However, research into sweeteners and appetite stimulation is inconsistent. Also, there is little evidence from longer-term studies to show that sweeteners lead to increased energy intake and contribute to the risk of obesity.

'While more research is needed, sweeteners continue to have a useful role in offering a sweet taste without adding extra calories,' says Carder.

1 April 2014

⇨ The above information is reprinted with kind permission from NHS Choices. Please visit www.nhs.uk for further information.

There's no debate: lowering salt cuts strokes and heart attacks

An article from The Conversation.

By Francesco Cappuccio, Cephalon Professor of Cardiovascular Medicine & Epidemiology at University of Warwick

THE CONVERSATION

The salt debate has filled the pages of health magazines and newspapers for years. From John Swales' original scepticism in 1988 to the Godlee's sharp call to reality in 1996, the debate has transcended the scientific arena into public opinion and media campaigns with increasingly passionate tones. Now a new study, published in *BMJ Open*, suggests that a 15% drop in daily salt intake in England between 2003 and 2011 led to 42% less stroke deaths and a 40% drop in deaths from coronary heart disease. So where does this leave the salt debate?

The salt controversy has been particularly heated since the translation of the results of scientific studies into public health and policy actions and the 'salt debate' has become for some a 'salt war'. The progression of this debate into a war resembles past and present debates (let us think about John Snow and the cholera epidemic in the 19th century, the long-lasting denial of the harm of tobacco smoking in the 20th century, global warming and climate change in the 21st century), when the translation of science into practice clashes with vested interests.

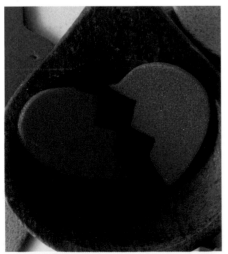

The scientific facts are: salt is causally related to blood pressure, the higher the salt intake, the higher the blood pressure, an effect seen since birth. A small reduction in salt intake (up to 50% of what we eat now) causes a fall in blood pressure in almost everyone across the whole range of blood pressure, although individuals will respond more or less, depending on factors like age, ethnicity, levels of blood pressure, body weight. High blood pressure causes strokes and heart attacks and a reduction in blood pressure reduces them. The effect is related to the size of the fall in blood pressure.

It is therefore conceivable that a moderate reduction in salt intake in a population would help reduce stroke and heart attacks through a reduction in blood pressure. The hypothesis is a no brainer but for scientists very difficult to 'prove'. To prove that a reduction of salt intake in populations over an extended period of time reduces the rate of strokes and heart attacks would need a randomised double-blind placebo-controlled clinical trial.

However, it has been argued that such a 'mother of trials' will never be possible. Should we then refrain from implementing public health policies based on the available evidence so far? A randomised clinical trial of tobacco smoking and lung cancer was never carried out in humans to 'prove' that smoking causes lung cancer and that we should eventually ban tobacco. And an assessment of the bulk of evidence underlying population action of salt reduction dwarfs the evidence that supports today-accepted policies on weight reduction, increase in physical exercise, intake of fibre, fruit and vegetable for the prevention of both cancer and cardiovascular disease.

The *BMJ Open* study is another contribution to the bulk of supportive evidence suggesting, though not proving, a plausible connection between the reduction in salt intake achieved in the last eight years in the UK with a national programme (1.4 g less salt per day) and the reduction of average population blood pressure (3.0/1.4 mmHg) and cardiovascular mortality (42% in stroke and 40% in ischaemic heart disease) during the same period.

The analysis used available datasets from repeated national surveys and indicates that the reduction in cardiovascular mortality was also compatible with a concomitant reduction in smoking, serum total cholesterol, and a modest increase in fruit and vegetable intake – but against a trend of a rise in average body weight.

Limitations are implicit in this type of analyses: ecological fallacy, unexplained confounding of the data and the use of crude mortality rates. The study probably will not satisfy those in need of hard science to prove population effects to support actions. However, it informs and encourages policy makers to the feasibility of implementing such programmes and the potential for small but significant sustained cost-saving effects.

15 April 2014

⇨ The above information is reprinted with kind permission from The Conversation. Please visit www.theconversation.com for further information.

Thousands of tonnes of saturated fat to be taken out of the nation's diet

More than one and a half Olympic-size swimming pools of saturated fat will be removed from the nation's diet over the next year as part of a drive to cut the amount of saturated fat in our food.

Almost half of the food manufacturing and retail industry has signed up to the Responsibility Deal 'Saturated Fat Reduction Pledge' by agreeing to reduce the amount of saturated fat in our food and change their products to make them healthier.

Cutting the amount of saturated fat we eat by just 15 per cent could prevent around 2,600 premature deaths every year from conditions such as cardiovascular disease, heart disease and stroke.

Public Health Minister, Jane Ellison said:

'One in six male deaths and one in nine female deaths are from coronary heart disease – this is why it's critical that we challenge the way we eat and that we all make changes where we can.

'It's hugely encouraging that companies providing almost half of the food available on the UK market have committed to this new Responsibility Deal pledge and they are leading the way to give their customers healthier products and lower fat alternatives.'

Some of the companies removing saturated fat from their products are:

⇨ Nestlé – which will remove 3,800 tonnes of saturated fat from over a billion Kit Kat bars per year by reformulating the recipe

⇨ Tesco – which will remove 32 tonnes of saturated fat from products such as breadsticks

⇨ Morrisons – which will be reformulating its spreads range to reduce saturated fat, this will remove approximately 50 tonnes

⇨ Aramark – which will increase the amount of one per cent fat milk it supplies across its sites and increase the training it gives to its chefs

⇨ Cricketer Farm – which will help one retailer remove 1.5 tonnes of saturated fat by switching to their half fat cheese.

Other companies that have pledged to make changes to their products are:

⇨ Subway – will reduce the amount of saturated fat in their Kids Pak™ by more than 70 per cent, replacing cookies and crisps with a healthier option which provides one of a child's recommended five-a-day portions of fruit and vegetables

⇨ Compass – which serves more than a million meals a day across their 7,000 sites, will be swapping to lower fat ingredients and promoting healthier menus as part of the pledge

⇨ Aldi – which will start a programme of saturated fat reformulation, explore reducing portion sizes and educating consumers and employees to choose healthier options

⇨ Sainsbury's – which will continue to reformulate recipes to reduce saturated fat

⇨ CH & Co – which will be reformulating some of its top-selling cakes

⇨ Unilever – which will continue to invest in spreads and blends that provide healthier options; in addition it will promote healthy eating by encouraging swaps in cooking and baking with lower saturated fat alternatives

⇨ Mondelez International – which will reformulate products across its portfolio, including BelVita, Oreo and Barny.

There are a number of ways that companies can lower the amount of saturated fat in our diets, including reformulating recipes so they include less fat, and introducing new products with lower fat.

Food and Drink Federation Director General, Melanie Leech said:

National Diet and Nutrition Survey – key findings: fat

Total fat: Mean total fat intake met the recommendation of no more than 35% food energy in all age/sex groups except for men aged 65 years and over, for whom, on average, total fat provided 36.0% food energy.

Saturated fat: Mean saturated fat intakes in all age groups exceeded the recommended level of no more than 11% food energy. For example, mean saturated fat intake for adults aged 19 to 64 years was 12.6% food energy.

Trans fat: Mean intakes of trans fat provided 0.7% of food energy for adults and older adults and 0.6% food energy for children, thus meeting the recommendation of no more than 2% food energy.

14 May 2014

Source: National Diet and Nutrition Survey: results from years 1, 2, 3 and 4 combined (2008/9 – 2011/12), 14 May 2014, Public Health England

'Today's announcement yet again underlines food and drink manufacturers' determination to play a full part in supporting improved public health.

'These significant commitments to reduce saturated fat in a wide range of products build on the achievements already delivered by a number of our members which empower consumers to make healthier choices appropriate for their lifestyles.'

The Responsibility Deal brings government and industry together to tackle public health issues and improve the health of the nation.

Chair of the Responsibility Deal Food Network, Professor Susan Jebb said:

'The Responsibility Deal has made great progress in changing our eating options and habits.

From the introduction of front of pack labelling to today's announcement, everyone involved can be proud of the work done so far – but we know more can be done.

These commitments to help reduce saturated fat are an important step forward. They recognise that too much saturated fat can increase cholesterol levels and cause heart disease and premature deaths which is why it's fantastic that so many companies have committed to helping people cut down on their consumption.

This development means we now have a suite of Responsibility Deal pledges that help companies cut fat, sugar and salt which together will help consumers achieve a healthier diet and reduce the risk of cardiovascular disease.'

26 October 2013

⇨ The above information is reprinted with kind permission from GOV.UK.

What is fat?

Fat is an essential part of our diet and nutrition, we cannot live without it.

Our bodies require small amounts of 'good fat' to function and help prevent disease. However, a lot of modern diets contain far more fat than the body needs. Too much fat, especially too much of the wrong type of fat, can cause serious health complaint including obesity, higher blood pressure and cholesterol levels, which in turn lead to a greater risk of heart disease.

Dietary fats make food tasty, they often improve the texture of food as well as flavour and smell – they make food more appealing. In the UK, the Department of Health suggests that no more than 35% of total calories should come from fat. In the US, recommended fat intake is 30% of total calorie intake. In reality most Western diets derive at least 40% (and sometimes a lot more) of their energy from fats.

Fat is good!

Like protein, but not carbohydrates, fat is essential to human life, we all need fat in our diets:

⇨ Fat is a concentrated source of energy – one gram of fat contains nine calories, much more than a gram of protein or carbohydrate which both contain four calories per gram. The body can pull on its fat reserves during lean times for energy, converting fat into glucose.

⇨ Fat provides a cushion to help protect our vital organs – without fat our organs would be more prone to damage. Furthermore, fat acts as an insulator, helping us to maintain the correct body temperature.

⇨ Fat enables our bodies to process vitamins A, D, E and K, which are all fat soluble and vital to good health.

⇨ Like amino acids in protein, fat contains essential fatty acids (EFAs). These EFAs are, as their name suggests, essential to good health and likely to help the heart and immune system. The human body cannot make its own (synthesise) these EFAs and therefore has to get them from consumption of fat.

⇨ Some fatty acids – like omega 3 – may provide other health benefits such as complementing the cognitive processes of the brain.

⇨ Fat makes food taste better. Hot buttered crumpets, double cream on trifle, gravy made from dripping!

Although we need fat we only need small quantities of the right kinds of fat to stay healthy. We all know that too much fat and consuming the wrong kind of fat can be detrimental to our health. (See 'Fat is bad' below).

Body Mass Index (BMI)

The term obese has become more commonplace in recent years. In the UK it is estimated that one in four adults is clinically obese – having a BMI of 30 or more. Obesity is, in most cases, caused by inappropriate diets, consuming too much fat.

To calculate your BMI:

Divide your weight in kilograms by the square of your height in metres.

Divide your weight in pounds by the square of your height in inches, and then multiply by 703.

The answer you get is your BMI:

If your BMI is less than 18.5 then you are underweight, you may need to gain weight.

If your BMI is between 18.5 and 24.9 you are an ideal weight.

If your BMI is between 25 and 29.9 you are classed as overweight and should take measures to lose weight.

If your BMI is over 30 then you are classed as obese. You should lose weight by changing your diet and/or increasing exercise.

BMI is not accurate in all cases – for example, people with athletic builds may have a high BMI – muscle is heavier than fat which can skew the results.

Fat is bad

Due to its high calorific value (1 gram of fat = 9 calories) it is easy to consume too many calories when eating fatty foods. Unused calories can be stored by the body as fat and will cause weight gain.

Our bodies store fat for lean times and have evolved to cope with seasonal availability of food – storing fat when food is plentiful and burning it off when food is scarce. In the modern world, and for most people, food is plentiful all year round – our bodies store fat but never burn it off, as fat accumulates we become overweight.

Fat can cushion and protect our internal organs; however, too much cushioning means more bulk and weight which in turn increases the workload of the heart and other organs.

Your body (the liver) produces cholesterol which is vital to a healthy body and a building block for other essential chemicals that the body produces. Cholesterol is a waxy substance that, in low levels, flows freely around your body in the blood. Higher levels of cholesterol mean a higher risk of developing coronary heart disease. See below for more on cholesterol.

Some fats are worse than others. Saturated fats are worse for you than unsaturated fats – this is to do with their chemical structure and how the body processes them. Trans or hydrogenated fats – which are almost exclusively manufactured (although do occur naturally in small quantities in meat and dairy produce) and are used in many processed foods – are particularly bad and are linked to an increased risk of high cholesterol levels and coronary heart disease.

Types of fat

Saturated and unsaturated

The two main types of fat are saturated and unsaturated. Unsaturated fats are generally considered better for us than saturated fats.

The reason that unsaturated fats are better is down to the molecular structure of fat. Saturated fat molecules form regular shapes that clump together easily; unsaturated fat molecules, however, form irregular shapes that cannot clump together so easily. Saturated fat is therefore more likely to stick to the sides of arteries and allow other saturated fat molecules to build up; this can gradually clog the arteries leading to higher blood pressure and making it more difficult for the heart to pump oxygen-rich blood around the body.

Fats are not soluble in water (or blood) and unless this problem is addressed – usually through change in diet and increased exercise – it can lead to serious health problems such as coronary heart disease.

Generally (although not exclusively) saturated fats come from animal sources (meat, dairy, eggs, etc.) and are usually solid at room temperature. Unsaturated fats come from vegetable sources (sunflower oil, olive oil, soya oil), oily fish (salmon, trout, mackerel, etc.) and soft margarines.

Vegetable sources do contain saturated fats but usually in low amounts; take oats for example, which contain almost 9% fat, made up of the three main types, saturated, monounsaturated and polyunsaturated.

Monounsaturated and polyunsaturated are the two main types of unsaturated fat – they are unsaturated as they are missing one (mono) or more (poly) hydrogen atoms in their chemical make-up – this is what gives them irregular shapes.

Hydrogenated or trans fat

Hydrogenated fat is manufactured fat used in processed foods. It contains some qualities desirable to food manufacturers, but is perhaps the worst of all fats when it comes to health.

Hydrogenated fat is vegetable fat that has been treated with extra hydrogen. This changes the chemical make-up of the fat – making it solid at room temperature. Technically, unsaturated fat, hydrogenated or trans-fat increases the risk of coronary heart disease by raising levels of LDL cholesterol and lowering levels of 'good' HDL cholesterol in the blood. This is the most important fat to avoid.

Cholesterol

Cholesterol is a type of fat found in the blood. Nearly all the cholesterol in the body is produced by the liver, very little is found in foods,

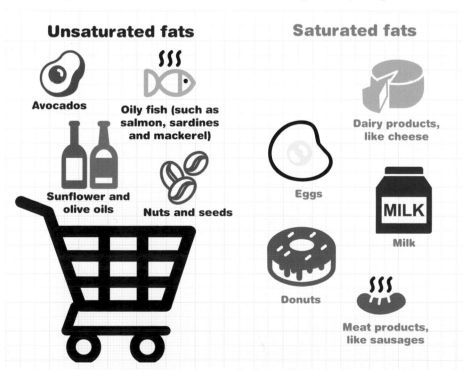

Unsaturated fats

Avocados

Oily fish (such as salmon, sardines and mackerel)

Sunflower and olive oils

Nuts and seeds

Saturated fats

Dairy products, like cheese

Eggs

MILK

Milk

Donuts

Meat products, like sausages

although seafood, liver, kidney and eggs do contain some cholesterol. Cholesterol is vital in the body, not only does it play a role in how all cells work but it is also a 'building block' for other essential chemicals that the body produces.

Cholesterol is carried around the body in the bloodstream combined with proteins, these are called lipoproteins. There are two main types of lipoprotein that are used to measure cholesterol levels in the blood.

Low-density lipoprotein (LDL) and High-density lipoprotein (HDL)

LDL is often called 'bad' cholesterol whereas HDL is considered 'good' cholesterol. HDL is 'good' as it can remove extra bad cholesterol from the bloodstream.

Blood cholesterol is measured by looking at the total LDL, HDL and other fats in the blood.

People with high cholesterol levels are more likely to develop health problems – the risks are increased further for people who also smoke, have high blood pressure, are physically inactive and unfit, are overweight or obese or suffer from diabetes.

A common cause of high cholesterol levels in modern society is the consumption of too much saturated fat.

Healthy fat tips

Read the labels of foods you buy. Try to reduce the amount of trans fats, hydrogenated fats and saturated fats in your diet – always favour foods with unsaturated fats.

If you are overweight then you should attempt to reduce your total fat intake – try to replace fatty foods with fresh fruit and vegetables. Increase your consumption of oily fish – omega 3 fats are known to provide many health benefits and most people do not consume enough – salmon, trout, fresh tuna and mackerel are all good.

⇨ The above information is reprinted with kind permission from SkillsYouNeed.com. Please visit www.skillsyouneed. com for further information.

About sugar

What is sugar?

Sugar is the naturally-occurring nutrient that makes food taste sweet. Sugar is a carbohydrate along with starch.

Carbohydrates are our main source of energy. Starch-rich foods include bread, rice, pasta, and potatoes, whereas sugars are found in fruit and vegetables, honey, jam and many soft drinks.

There are a number of different sugars:

⇨ Glucose and fructose are found in fruit and vegetables

⇨ Milk sugar is known as lactose

⇨ Maltose (malt sugar) is found in malted drinks and beer

⇨ Sucrose comes from sugar cane or beet and is often referred to as 'table' or 'added' sugar. It also occurs naturally in some fruit and vegetables.

These different types of sugar have the same nutritional value.

⇨ Starches and sugars provide about four calories per gram.

⇨ A level teaspoon of sugar (4 g) provides 16 calories.

Nutrition experts worldwide recommend that adults and children above the age of two obtain at least 50% of their daily calories from a variety of carbohydrate sources.

Eating sugar is a useful way of increasing carbohydrate intake especially in those with high energy requirements, such as athletes and people employed in physically demanding jobs.

Most people eat starchy foods in combination with fat, e.g. butter with bread, creamy sauce with pasta, potatoes fried in oil. However, sugar itself is fat-free, and per gram, contains less than half the calories of fat.

Types and uses

Different types of sugar

The most obvious difference between types of sugars used in the home is colour. When sugar has been extracted from the juice of the beet or cane plant, a strong tasting black syrup (known as molasses) remains. When white sugar is made, the molasses are entirely removed, whereas brown sugars retain varying amounts of this natural syrup. The more molasses in brown sugar, the stickier the crystals, the darker the colour and the stronger

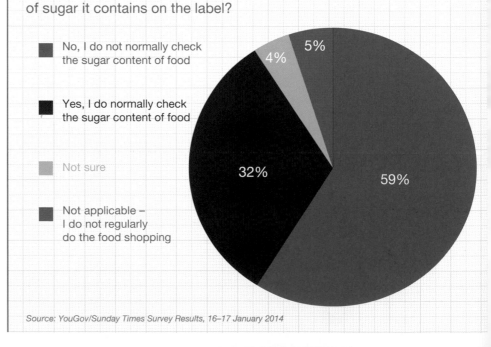

When buying food, do you normally check the amount of sugar it contains on the label?

- No, I do not normally check the sugar content of food
- Yes, I do normally check the sugar content of food
- Not sure
- Not applicable – I do not regularly do the food shopping

5%
4%
32%
59%

Source: YouGov/Sunday Times Survey Results, 16–17 January 2014

the flavour. However, the presence of molasses does not change sugar's nutritional value.

As well as differences in colour and flavour, sugars vary in the size of their crystals:

⇨ **Granulated:** all-purpose sugar for general use ('table' sugar)

⇨ **Caster:** small grains ensure smooth blending to give even textures in cakes and other baked foods

⇨ **Icing:** dissolves very quickly because of its very fine texture – useful for decorating cakes.

Uses of sugar

⇨ **As a sweetener:** sugar is added to foods or drinks to make them taste more pleasant. For example, it balances the bitterness of coffee or reduces the tartness of sour fruit.

⇨ **As a preservative:** sugar is a natural preservative that binds water to prevent the growth of micro-organisms, thereby reducing food spoilage, as in jams and preserves.

⇨ **As a bulking agent:** sugars give texture to a variety of foods from jams to frozen products.

Sugar makes food taste good

We are born with a liking for sweetness, and most people continue to enjoy sweet foods throughout their lifetime. It would be a pity to forget that eating is also about pleasure!

Sugar improves the flavour of foods, and so widens the range of foods that people will eat. Without sugar, for example, many high-fibre breakfast cereals providing important nutrients would be inedible. Sour and bitter fruits also taste much better when sugar is added.

An expert committee report (FAO, 1998) commented: 'Moderate intake of sugar-rich foods can also provide for a palatable and nutritious diet.'

⇨ The above information is reprinted with kind permission from Sugar Nutrition UK. Please visit www.sugarnutrition.org.uk for further information.

© Sugar Nutrition UK

Sugars in ingredients

When looking at an ingredients list you may see different sugars listed. The name that is used in this is dictated by legal requirements. Below are the most common sugars and sources of sugars that you may come across:

Glucose (dextrose)	A monosaccharide (single sugar) that is found in plants. It is in fruit and vegetables and can be used in foods such as biscuits and cereal bars.
Fructose	A monosaccharide that is also found primarily in fruit and vegetables. It can be added to food products such as sports drinks and bars.
Lactose	A milk sugar found in dairy products. It can also be an ingredient in foods like biscuits and instant soups.
Sucrose (table sugar)	A disaccharide (two joined sugars) made up of glucose and fructose. Found in plants – it is present in sugar beet, sugar cane, fruit and vegetables. It can be an ingredient in foods such as cakes, biscuits and drinks. It is also the type of sugar that we buy in the shops called granulated, caster, demerara, etc. These packets of sugar are the sucrose extracted from either sugar beet or sugar cane.
Maltose	A disaccharide made up of two glucose molecules. It is found in germinating seeds such as barley and is used in malted drinks and beers.
Isoglucose (glucose-fructose syrup)	Made from hydrolysed starch, this is comprised of approximately 58% glucose and 42% fructose. This can be used in cakes, cereals, fruit products and drinks.
Invert sugar	A mixture of glucose and fructose, obtained from the hydrolysis of sucrose and found in fruits and honey. It can be used in foods like confectionery, ice-cream and baked foods.
Honey	Made by bees as food for the hive, this contains fructose and glucose. With its unique taste it can be an ingredient in foods such as snack bars and cakes.
Molasses/ treacle	A viscous syrup that is a by-product of extracting sucrose. This contains sucrose, glucose and fructose and can be used in foods such as gingerbread.
Agave syrup	Extracted from the agave plant, this primarily contains fructose and some glucose. It can be used as an ingredient in products such as drinks, confectionery and cakes.
Fruit juice concentrates	Concentrated fruit juices provide a source of fructose, glucose and sucrose. These can come from a wide range of different fruits, so can be called, for example, grape, date or prune syrup. These can be used to sweeten drinks, biscuits, cakes, etc.
High-Fructose Corn Syrup (HFCS)	This comprises of fructose and glucose, extracted from corn. Although this receives a lot of media attention and is a common product in America, it is not commonly used in the UK.

FactCheck: is sugar really bad for you?

The claim

'It's calories that count when it comes to weight loss, not uniquely calories from sugar.'

American Beverage Association statement

The background

Sugar is becoming the big dietary villain of our times.

We used to think it was saturated fat that made us fat. But fat consumption fell and we carried on getting more obese and unwell.

All those low-fat products on the supermarket shelves just happen to be full of added sugar.

A swelling chorus of doctors and dieticians are now warning that the white stuff is the real culprit, leading to higher rates of diabetes and other illness as well as expanding waistlines.

Last week the World Health Organization (WHO) recommended people halve their sugar intake.

Is this just another fad that will be replaced by another dietary bogeyman, or is it really time to yank out our sweet tooth?

The analysis

The food industry is at war with a very vocal group of campaigners on the issue of whether we should restrict or tax sugary foods.

The big question is whether it's fair to pick on sugar. Are we eating too much generally, taking in too many calories from fat or starch or sugar or whatever, or is there something particularly bad about sugar?

Big Food's position on this could not be clearer.

The industry-funded World Sugar Research Organisation (WRSO) says: 'Over-consumption of food energy, whatever its macronutrient composition, and inadequate physical activity may lead to body weight gain and increase risk of Type 2 DM (diabetes mellitus).'

Coca-Cola says: 'All calories count, no matter where they come from.'

The American Beverage Association: 'It's calories that count when it comes to weight loss, not uniquely calories from sugar.'

Get the idea?

Anti-sugar campaigners are equally adamant that there is something especially bad about sugar and we need to single it out for attention.

General advice about getting less calories overall and more exercise just won't cut it.

There is surprisingly little medical research that gets to the crux of this question.

In order to isolate the effect of sugar we need to get two groups of people

to eat the same amount of total calories, but vary the amount of sugar within the diets, then track the results.

Large-scale, long-term studies of this kind are few and far between.

Before it issued its recent draft guidance on sugar, the WHO commissioned a review of the evidence on sugar intake and body weight, published in the *British Medical Journal* last year.

The conclusions are actually very cautious, with the authors finding 'rapid weight gain that occurs after an increased intake of sugars' but concluding that 'the extent to which population-based advice to reduce sugars might reduce risk of obesity cannot be extrapolated from the present findings'.

The team found 12 studies which kept total calories the same but varied sugar intake, swapping sugar for more complex carbohydrates like bread and potatoes in one group.

They 'saw no evidence of difference in weight change as a result of differences in sugars intakes when energy intakes were equivalent'.

The researchers added: 'The data suggest that the change in body fatness that occurs with modifying intake of sugars results from an alteration in energy balance rather than a physiological or metabolic consequence of (simple sugars).'

It's possible to see this as a victory for the food industry – a validation of what they have been saying all along.

But this isn't the end of the story.

These studies limited participants to a predetermined number of calories a day, something not representative of reality outside the laboratory.

What if eating a lot of sugar makes it harder for you to limit your overall calorie intake in real life?

Some doctors have suggested that sugary soft drinks are associated with weight gain because of their 'low satiety'.

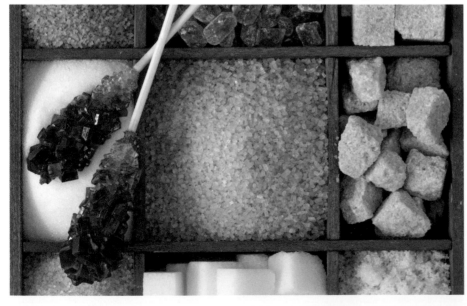

In other words, you don't feel full after guzzling a can of cola, even though you've taken hundreds of calories on board, and you eat just as much later.

Others say sugar may be physically addictive, acting on the brain in the same way drugs like cocaine do, but most positive evidence comes from experiments on lab rats, not humans.

Dr Robert Lustig, an American paediatrician at the forefront of the campaign against sugar, says the body reacts differently to sugar than other foods.

His theory is that sugar causes a unique spike in the hormone insulin, which tells the body to store fat and blocks another hormone that tells us when we are full.

When he gives obese children a drug to reduce the insulin response, they start eating less and losing weight.

The theory has some supporters among doctors but remains controversial.

So far we have been talking about weight gain and obesity, but new research suggests sugar carries other dangers besides an expanding waistline.

Last year a US study using long-term data from 175 countries found an association between the availability of sugar in a population's food supply and rates of type 2 diabetes.

The trend was independent of obesity rates and a host of other possible confounding factors.

Increasing sugar by 150 calories per person per day was correlated with a one per cent increase in the prevalence of diabetes in a country's population.

An extra 150 calories of any other type increased the diabetes rate by just 0.1 per cent.

Another US study published last month found a significant relationship between eating more added sugar and the risk of dying from heart disease.

Again, this was independent of body mass and index physical activity.

The verdict

The sugar industry maintains that excess calories are the problem, not excess sugar.

Purely on the issue of weight gain, it's interesting to note that the very researchers commissioned by the WHO before it updated its sugar guidelines actually tentatively back the industry on this point.

That doesn't mean sugar is off the hook. It means more evidence is needed to settle the point one way or the other.

New research linking sugar with diabetes and heart disease is interesting and the industry has not come up with an answer to it yet.

The WHO has added its voice to the growing number of doctors who have decided that there is enough evidence of various health risks to start advising people to cut down on sugar now.

14 March 2014

⇨ The above information is reprinted with kind permission from Channel 4. Please visit www.channel4.com for further information.

Soft Drinks Survey 2014

Product name	Flavour	Sugars/100 g	Sugars/330 ml* serving	Teaspoons sugar equiv/330 ml* serving
Old Jamaica Ginger Beer with Extra Fiery Jamaica Root Ginger	Ginger beer	15.7	52	13
Club Orange 2 litres	Orange	14.3	47	12
Sainsbury's Cloudy Lemonade	Lemonade	13.5	45	11
Tesco Fiery Ginger Beer	Ginger Beer	13.3	44	11
Cherry Coca-Cola 2 litres	Flavoured Cola	11.2	37	9
7UP 1.25 litres	Lemonade	11.2	37	9
Tesco Classic Cola 2 litres	Cola	10.9	36	9
Barr Irn Bru	Other	10.5	35	9
Dr Pepper 2 litres	Cola	10.4	34	9
Lidl Freeway Orange	Orange	10	33	8
Fanta Orange 500 ml	Orange	6.9	23	6
Asda Chosen by You Dandelion & Burdock 2 litres	Dandelion & Burdock	6.8	22	6
Asda Chosen by You Iron Brew 2 litres	Other	4	13	3
The Co-operative Lemonade 2 litres	Lemonade	1	3	1

Product information was collected online, instore or direct from manufacturers.

*Serving size has been standardised to 330 ml, regular can size. The survey was carried out between 1 and 30 May 2014 and products checked week commencing 2 June 2014. *Source: Soft Drinks Survey 2014, Action on Sugar, 2014*

'Sugar tax' proposed by campaign group to curb child obesity

Campaign group, Action on Sugar has created a strategy document of seven critical areas of policy to prevent childhood obesity in the UK, which it has presented to Jeremy Hunt MP, Secretary of State for Health this month – which includes the introduction of a sugar tax.[1]

Action on Sugar is a group of specialists concerned with sugar and its effects on health. With one in five ten to 11-year-olds now obese and one in three overweight, the Action on Sugar plan details the following key actions to change the food environment, which is responsible for the obesity epidemic:[2]

⇨ Reduce added sugars by 40% by 2020 by reformulating food[3]

⇨ Cease all forms of targeted marketing of ultra-processed, unhealthy foods and drinks to children

⇨ Disassociate physical activity with obesity via banning junk food sports sponsorships

⇨ Reduce fat in ultra-processed foods, particularly saturated fat – 15% reduction by 2020

⇨ Limit the availability of ultra-processed foods and sweetened soft drinks as well as reducing portion size

⇨ Incentivise healthier food and discourage drinking of soft drinks by introducing a sugar tax

⇨ Remove responsibility for nutrition from the Department of Health and return it back to an independent agency.

If these actions are followed, Action on Sugar says the UK Government will be the first country in the world to halt the obesity epidemic by reducing calories by 100 kcal a day.[4] At present, the costs of obesity and type 2 diabetes are estimated at approximately £29 billion a year, and given the number of children who are now obese, this figure is predicted to rise exponentially. The direct and indirect costs of treating type 2 diabetes alone are predicted to rise from £21.8 billion to £35.6 billion by 2035.[5]

Professor Graham MacGregor, Chairman of Action on Sugar says: 'Obesity in children leads to the premature development of cardiovascular disease, stroke, heart attacks and heart failure, which are the commonest cause of death and disability in the UK. Obesity predisposes to type 2 diabetes, which further increases the risk of cardiovascular disease and also, importantly, it can lead to severe complications, i.e. the commonest cause of blindness, renal dialysis and amputation of the lower limbs. These complications are extremely expensive to manage, and will cripple the NHS if the increase in obesity and type 2 diabetes is not stopped immediately.'

Dr Aseem Malhotra, Cardiologist and Science Director of Action on Sugar says: 'It is really quite shameful that the food industry continues to spend billions in junk food advertising targeting children, the most vulnerable members of society. They even manage to associate sugary products with sport. Physical activity has a multitude of benefits but a child doing an hour of PE every day would be putting all to waste if they ended up gorging on a burger and chips and a packet of crisps washed down with a sugary drink. One has to run half a marathon to burn off those calories. It's time to bust the myth of physical activity and obesity and dissociate junk food and sport.'

23 June 2014

⇨ The above information is reprinted with kind permission from Patient.co.uk. Please visit www.patient.co.uk for further information.

1 Childhood Obesity Action Plan

2 Jebb SA. Dietary determinants of obesity. Obesity reviews : an official journal of the International Association for the Study of Obesity 2007;8 Suppl 1:93

3 ... Brinsden and G A MacGregor, 2013. ... the United Kingdom: a successful ... health. http://www.nature.com/ ...ent/abs/jhh2013105a.html

4 Department of Health, 2011. Healthy lives, healthy people. https://www.gov.uk/government/uploads/system/uploads/attachment_data/file/213720/dh_130487.pdf.

5 Diabetic Medicine: http://www.diabetes.org.uk/About_us/News_Landing_Page/NHS-spending-on-diabetes-to-reach-169-billion-by-2035 /

Why sugar isn't the bad guy

By Ian Mellis

Just as fat was demonised in the 1980s sugar seems to be taking a bashing as dietary zealots, whipping boy. With sugar avoidance becoming the latest media headline it's compelling that sugar now plays the role that saturated fat once played and it is now responsible for the obesity epidemic that was once fat's responsibility.

With what has been published you never really hear about the positive side of sugar or how it is used in the human body. Overwhelmingly, the opinion of newspapers and numerous documentaries is that sugar is evil incarnate and will get you addicted, hooked on the giddy feeling of euphoria that only milk chocolate can give before you are sat in a pile of high-sugar energy drinks looking for your next hit if you can get your obese frame out of bed.

The alarmism highlights that sugar correlates with a number of diseases from diabetes, hypertension and heart disease. However, all of these conditions are multi-factorial in cause. You cannot attribute their development purely to sugar intake. Lifestyle and other dietary behaviours are also responsible.

What also is clear is that over the last 30 years activity has decreased as we undertake more sedentary occupations while total calorific intake

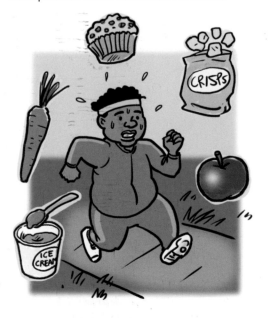

has increased by over 400 calories daily. Sugar consumption, although being blamed for the increase in people's weight, has only risen by a few calories on average since the 1970s. In fact the consumption of fats, oils, dairy fats and flour and cereal products have increased by about 180 calories which is about 4.5 times the average increase in the intake of sugar. In summation, we are not eating excessively more sugar than what we were consuming 30 years ago.

This point highlights that modern lifestyles indicate we are eating more of everything and we are less active than the previous generation. It's a bit hard then to primarily blame sugar for this issue as we do not see an exact change in sugar consumption in line with weight gain.

Let's look at sugar's role in the body. All things will kill you if you over consume them – sugar included. So will water, but the volumes needed to be consumed for it to be poisonous to end your life are pretty extreme. A 200-pound man would need to consume six pounds of pure sugar to kill himself. While I agree that there are negatives about overconsumption of sugar there are negatives about overconsumption of everything – sugar therefore is as poisonous as water, should this be the media story – I am not too sure?

Sugar is one of our main sources of energy when broken down in to glycogen. We hold about 350 g of muscle glycogen, 90 g in the liver and about 5 g circulating in our blood. We replenish it when we eat. Predominantly we break sugar down from carbohydrates (not just sugars) so grains, potatoes, vegetables, pasta and rice among other sources provide our dietary intake to keep us well stocked up on energy. Sugar is just classified as a carbohydrate – we evolved to use sugars as an energy source; completely ignoring it as a way of producing energy you could argue is like driving a car with three wheels –

it's possible but it's not exactly going to be a comfy ride.

When we consume carbohydrates, insulin is elevated (this will depend upon the type of food consumed and what it is consumed with). Insulin is associated with driving energy towards storage and hence it has an association with an increase in stored fat. This twinned with the lack of production associated with 'over production' being a symptom of type 2 diabetes.

This is where the correlation of high sugar equals high insulin resulting in high body fat comes from. That may be the case if you walk around eating sugar all day or eating an excessive amount of carbohydrates for prolonged periods where insulin is chronically elevated.

Guess what, though insulin is only elevated post feeding in healthy individuals, your body stores fat as well when insulin is low, elevated insulin suppresses your appetite and those of you who thought you were safe on your high-protein diet, guess what? Protein stimulates insulin increase. Sugar or carbohydrates have been demonised but simply the science is not there as correlation does not necessitate cause especially when you look at the sugar/elevated insulin/fat gain hypothesis.

'What is a healthy sugar intake?' is perhaps the most prudent question. In our pursuit of dietary fads we have completely lost sight of what is enough and what is excessive. In my next post I will discuss what is sensible and what is excessive and why the term 'natural' sugar really does not mean anything.

3 March 2014

⇨ Ian Mellis is the owner of Results FAST (www.resultsfast.co.uk) a fitness and nutrition training centre based in Ware, Hertfordshire. For more information contact info@resultsfast.co.uk.

© Ian Mellis 2014

Any defence of sugar is pure confection

More and more people are challenging the food industry's PR machine. The evidence shows that sugar, not fat, is the enemy.

By Aseem Malhotra

The Public Health Minister, Anna Soubry, has commented that the poor are more likely to be obese. It is well known that social status is linked to health, but her comments were also motivated by a mentality that victimises the most vulnerable. She should really be directing her criticism at the food industry. There is no doubt that an oversupply of cheap junk food fuelled by unregulated and irresponsible marketing limits our ability to make healthy choices. But there is an equally important question that merits attention: are we being given the wrong dietary advice?

A patient recently came to see me for a cardiovascular evaluation. He was particularly baffled as to why he had gained a stone in weight several months after he had followed a dietician's instructions to lower his blood cholesterol by eating 'low fat' products. How could this have happened?

This week the *British Medical Journal*'s front page asked: 'Is sugar the real culprit in the obesity epidemic?', a response to a study published in the same edition that concluded that cutting sugar intake led to significant weight loss. A paediatric endocrinologist, Professor Robert Lustig, has highlighted the toxic, addictive and appetite-driving properties of sugar. His 90-minute lecture has attracted worldwide attention with over three million views on YouTube. But the dangers of sugar is not news to the scientific community. A British professor and nutritionist, John Yudkin, believed that sugar, not fat, was the biggest culprit in heart disease and in 1972 set this out in his book, *Pure, White and Deadly*.

Research has moved on a great deal, and recent research has revealed that saturated fat from dairy products in particular may actually be protective against heart disease and stroke. Dairy products are exemplary providers of Vitamin A and D in which many British people are deficient. Calcium and phosphorus, also found in dairy products, may be beneficial to health through blood pressure-lowering effects. Vitamin D deficiency has been strongly associated with cardiovascular death.

Highly processed foods advertised as 'low fat' are often loaded with cheaply added excess sugars and preservatives. Cereals and flavoured yoghurts are just a few examples. I have started to advise my patients to eat butter instead of margarine and just eat real food. But even doctors' own dietary beliefs are strongly influenced by industry advertising. I was recently surprised to discover that there was no scientific basis to the heavily promoted claims made on behalf of a well-known sports drink that I had been taking on my daily visits to the gym – that it has performance-enhancing qualities. Instead of wasting £7,000 in the past 15 years buying a product loaded with sugar, I would have been better off drinking tap water.

There is universal scientific consensus that trans fats found in fast food and processed foods such as biscuits, crisps and frozen pizza are detrimental to health and may even increase the short-term risk of a heart attack. The British Medical Association has rightly called for a reduction of trans fats, salt and sugar in pre-prepared foods.

And as to 'saturated fat' and weight gain? Professor David Haslam, chair of the National Obesity Forum, says that all calories are not created equal. 'It's extremely naive of the public and the medical profession to imagine that a calorie of bread, a calorie of meat and a calorie of alcohol are all dealt in the same way by the amazingly complex systems of the body. The assumption has been made that increased fat in the bloodstream is caused by increased saturated fat in the diet, whereas modern scientific evidence is proving that refined carbohydrates and sugar in particular are actually the culprits.'

Big tobacco was able to stall government intervention by planting doubt in relation to smoking and lung cancer for half a century and 'big food' continues to deny that sugar is harmful. The academic vice president of the Royal College of Physicians, John Wass, is right to suggest that medical students should have more lectures on nutrition. But the advice doctors give when dealing with overweight patients should be based upon the best available scientific evidence, not what the food industry wants us to believe. As an isolated voice, Yudkin, who died in 1995, may have lost the battle with the sugar industry four decades ago, but big food will find it more difficult to silence his growing army of disciples whose only incentive is to expose what's right for public health.

24 January 2013

⇨ The above information is reprinted with kind permission from *The Guardian*. Please visit www.theguardian.com for further information.

Chapter 2

Make healthier choices

Tips for a healthier diet

Eating a healthy diet will make you feel better, give you more energy and boost your immune system. It will also help prevent certain illnesses and diseases.

This Bank Workers Charity guide shows 20 ways you can start to make changes to your diet so that you can develop a healthier way of eating. You can also find sources of further information at the end.

Eat the right amount

If you eat more calories than you burn off, this will accumulate as fat. Doing this on a regular basis can lead to obesity which can increase the risk of type 2 diabetes, heart disease and some cancers. Exactly how much you need to eat each day will depend on how active you are and on your size but the general rule of thumb is that men need 2,500 calories a day and women need 2,000. Ways of limiting the number of calories you eat are:

⇨ to reduce your portion size

⇨ to refuse second helpings

⇨ to eat from a smaller plate

⇨ to avoid supersize portions when eating out

⇨ to opt for lower calorie foods, such as choosing to snack on a piece of fruit rather than eating a bag of crisps or a chocolate bar.

Eat five portions of fruit and vegetables a day

Eating fruit and vegetables is essential for a healthy diet as they contain vitamins, minerals and fibre as well as phyto-nutrients which act as antioxidants to protect the body from harmful free radicals. All fruit and vegetables are beneficial but choose those that are bright or dark in colour (such as red peppers, beetroot, blueberries and tomatoes) as they contain higher quantities of nutrients. Another important group is the brassica family, which includes broccoli, cabbage, cauliflower, curly kale and sprouts.

Try to eat fruit and vegetables at every mealtime and as a snack in between meals. Also, try to eat them raw as the cooking process destroys many of the vitamins and minerals. When you do cook them, steam them rather than boil them.

What is a portion?

A portion of fresh fruit or vegetables is 80 g.

That equates to:

⇨ one piece of fruit you can hold in your hand (e.g. an apple, pear, banana, orange)

⇨ three apricots

⇨ a handful of grapes

⇨ a bowl of vegetable soup

⇨ three sticks of celery

⇨ a slice of melon or pineapple

⇨ half a grapefruit

⇨ a side salad

⇨ three tablespoons of beans, peas or sweetcorn

⇨ two broccoli spears.

A portion of dried fruit is 30 g which is around one heaped tablespoon of raisins, currants and sultanas or three prunes.

A portion of fruit juice or vegetable juice is a 150 ml glass.

Eat whole grains

Opt for whole grains such as wholemeal bread, porridge, whole grain cereals and pasta, brown rice, oatcakes and rye bread. Try to reduce refined grains such as white bread, white pasta and white rice as these have had much of the fibre and nutrients stripped from them.

Eat more fibre

Fibre keeps your digestive system healthy, lowers cholesterol and helps you feel fuller for longer. It is found in fruit, vegetables and whole grains. You need to aim for about 18 g of fibre a day – see the packaging for guidelines on the amounts of fibre the food contains.

Eat foods rich in calcium

Calcium helps to build strong bones and teeth. Aim to eat foods rich in calcium, such as dairy products (milk, yoghurt, cheese, fromage frais), dark green leafy vegetables (especially watercress), almonds and sesame seeds. Some drinks (such as soya milk) are fortified with calcium, so opt for these if you do not eat much dairy.

Eat protein

We need to eat protein on a daily basis for the growth and repair of our bodies. It is found in meat, fish, eggs, nuts, seeds, pulses (lentils, beans and peas) and soya.

Due to the high levels of saturated fat in red meat, opt for white meat (such as turkey or chicken) and fish. Most people in the Western world eat too much protein; you only need a couple of servings a day. For example, one serving is 100 g of meat or fish or two eggs.

Eat more fish

Try to eat fish at least twice a week, which includes one portion of oily fish (salmon, mackerel, sardines, pilchards, anchovies, herring or fresh tuna – not canned). Fish contains protein, vitamins and minerals and oily fish has omega 3 fats which may help prevent heart disease.

Cut down on sugary foods

Sugary foods, such as sweets and confectionery, jams, puddings, biscuits, cakes and fizzy drinks are high in calories, low in nutrients and bad for your teeth, so should be avoided. If you have a sweet tooth and find it hard to give these up, buy artificially sweetened or reduced sugar foods. Drink fruit juice or water instead of sugary drinks and eat a piece of fruit which contains natural sugars rather than a chocolate bar or cake.

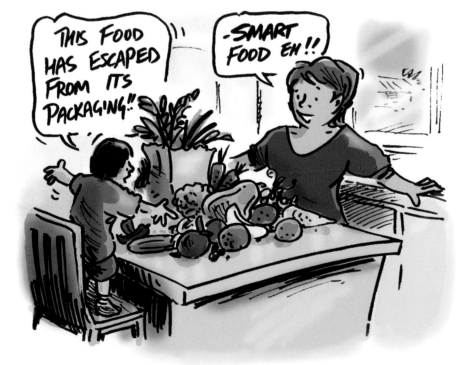

Cut down on salt

Too much salt can lead to high blood pressure, fluid retention or breathing difficulties. Aim to have no more than 6 g a day which is a rounded teaspoon. To reduce your intake, cut down on ready meals and processed foods as these contain higher levels of salt. Try to avoid those foods with red salt 'traffic light' labels altogether. Other ways of cutting down are to not add salt to your food (either when cooking it or when on your plate), to rinse canned vegetables and to buy reduced-salt foods.

Cut down on saturated fat

Saturated fat can increase cholesterol levels which can lead to heart disease. It is found in butter, lard, cream and cheese as well as those foods made with saturated fat, such as pastries, cakes, biscuits, pies and ice cream. Meat fat is also saturated fat so try to cut the fat off when you eat meat and buy lean mince. Buy skimmed or semi-skimmed milk, low fat yoghurt and reduced fat spread. Avoid creamy sauces, food fried in butter or lard and battered fish. Always read labels on ready meals and go for products with a green saturated fat traffic light label.

Opt for unsaturated fat

It is important to eat fat as part of your diet as it provides energy and aids the absorption of certain vitamins. However, opt for unsaturated fats which are 'healthy' fats as they will help protect the cardiovascular system and hydrate the skin.

Unsaturated fats can be found in oily fish, nuts, vegetable oils and soft margarine. Omega-3 fatty acids in fish oil also have anti-inflammatory properties and can reduce joint pain.

Cut down on processed foods

Smoked, cured and processed foods such as smoked ham, bacon, sausages, salami, pepperoni and garlic sausage contain added salt and tend to be higher in saturated fat as well. Try to limit the amounts of this kind of food.

Cut down on caffeine

Caffeine is a stimulant that can lead to increased blood pressure. It is found in tea, coffee, cola, chocolate and energy drinks. Limit the number of such drinks or go for decaffeinated versions.

Do not skip breakfast

Eating breakfast will provide you with energy first thing and will help you from getting an energy dip mid morning when it is tempting to eat sugary snacks. For breakfast, aim to eat whole grain cereal or whole wheat toast with eggs, as well as a piece of fruit or fruit juice.

Drink plenty of fluids

Water helps flush out our systems and is essential for our survival. Aim to drink between six to eight glasses of fluid a day to keep you hydrated. Fruit juice, milk, coffee and tea count towards this. Alcoholic drinks do not. You will need more liquids during hot weather and after exercising. Not drinking enough will result in headaches or tiredness.

Reduce your alcohol intake

Too much alcohol will damage your liver, affecting its ability to function properly. Try to limit your intake to 21 units a week for men and 14 for women, with two alcohol-free days per week. A unit is half a pint of beer, a 175 ml glass of wine or one pub measure of sherry, spirit or liqueur. Alcohol is high in calories (a pint of beer and a large glass of wine have almost 200 calories) so limiting your intake will also help you moderate your weight.

Get the right balance

There are five main food groups: carbohydrates (starchy food such as bread, potatoes, rice and pasta); fruit and vegetables; dairy; meat, fish, eggs and beans; and foods containing fat and sugar.

The 'eatwell plate' will help you get the right balance of each group. Minimise the amount of saturated fat and sugar but do not cut out any other groups, such as carbohydrates.

Do not deny yourself

Eating a healthier diet does not mean you have to deprive yourself of your favourite foods. For example, telling yourself you can never eat crisps again will only make you crave them more. Indulging in the occasional 'banned' food is fine, as long as you do not eat a large amount of it or eat it too often.

Eat a variety of foods

The key to a balanced diet is to eat a wide range of foods, so that you get the vitamins and nutrients you need. So, rather than buy the same items in your weekly shop, go for variety. For example, when making a salad or stir fry, try to include as many vegetables as you can and aim for a 'rainbow' effect of different colours.

Learn how to change your eating habits

If you know your diet is unhealthy and you eat too many sugary, fatty and processed foods and not enough fruit, vegetables and whole grains, it will probably be difficult to make the sudden change to eating healthily.

Start by making a conscious effort to introduce small changes and, in time, this will become a habit. Here are some ways you can add healthier choices to your daily diet:

⇨ Grill meat and fish rather than fry it.

⇨ Pour tomato-based sauces over pasta, rather than cheesy, creamy sauces.

⇨ Mash potatoes in skimmed milk rather than butter.

⇨ Read labels on foods so you are aware of the salt, fat and sugar contents.

⇨ Eat boiled eggs with wholemeal toast for breakfast, not fried eggs and bacon.

⇨ Order a skinny latte at your local coffee shop.

⇨ Buy unsalted nuts.

⇨ Top your baked potato with baked beans or cottage cheese instead of grated cheese.

⇨ Eat porridge, not sugary cereals.

⇨ Have some dried fruit and seeds as a mid-afternoon snack instead of a slice of cake.

⇨ Swap your bag of crisps in your lunchbox for a salad.

⇨ Aim to replace one meal of red meat each week with chicken, turkey or fish.

Further information

BBC – for information on nutrition and balancing your diet.

NHS – for information, recipes and online tools on healthy eating.

Department of Health – for government updates on food and nutrition news.

December 2012

⇨ The above information is reprinted with kind permission from the Bank Workers Charity. Please visit www.bwcharity.org.uk for further information.

Understanding food labels

With increasing rates of overweight/obesity worldwide, we are forever being told to follow a healthy diet and that homemade is usually best. Unfortunately, due to work/study, family or other pressures and time constraints, convenience has a big influence on our food choices. It is in these situations especially that understanding how to read food labels is important.

1. Nutrition labels can help you

⇨ Compare products/brands

⇨ Check how much fat, sugar or salt is in a food

⇨ Choose the healthiest option

⇨ Check the ingredients

⇨ Understand what a typical portion size is

2. What am I looking for?

Average adult guidelines:

⇨ Female = 2000 kcal per day

⇨ Male = 2500 kcal per day

3. I need to make a quick decision!

⇨ Some labels use red, amber and green (traffic light) colour coding

⇨ A quick glance can help you discover whether a food is high, medium or low in calories, sugar, fat, saturated fat and salt

● **High**
● Medium
● **Low**

⇨ Generally, the more green lights, the healthier the choice!

4. The ingredients list

⇨ Ingredients are listed in order of weight (main ingredients first)

⇨ Look out for various names for sugar, e.g. high-fructose corn syrup, sucrose, dextrose, glucose, maltose and fructose... they can quickly add up!

⇨ If there is a long list of ingredients this may indicate that the product is highly processed or contains added flavourings and preservatives. Is there a more natural alternative?

⇨ The above information, and the figure below, are reprinted with kind permission from Loughborough University. Please visit www.lboro.ac.uk for further information.

© Loughborough University 2014

Average adult guidelines:
Female = 2000 kcal/d
Male = 2500 kcal/d

Always compare nutrition information 'per 100 g', not per portion, as these may differ.

Don't be misled by claims. Sometimes a reduction reduction in fat can mean more sugar, sweeteners or other added ingredients.

How much energy you need will depend on your age, gender & physical activity levels.

High sugar = more than 15 g per 100 g

Low fat = less than 3/1.5 g per 100 g for solid/liquid foods, respectively.

High saturated fat more than 5 g per

'Light/Lite' means that it contains at least 30% less (fat/calories/sugar) than standard products.

Don't be enticed by bright, fancy packaging – try to look closer at the label!

You can also find the nutrient content of many restaurant/fast food meals online!

Spinach & ricotta pizza

Typical values (cooked as per instructions)	Per 100g	Per 1/2 pizza	% based on GDA for ….	Women	Men
Energy	1001 kJ 238 kcal	1977 kJ 470 kcal	23.5%	2000 kcal	2500 kcal
Protein	9.3g	18.4g	40.9%	45g	55g
Carbohydrate	28.7g	56.7g	24.7%	230g	300g
of which sugars	2.7g	5.3g	5.9%	90g	120g
of which starch	25.9g	51.2g	-	-	-
Fat	9.6g	19.0g	27.1%	70g	95g
of which saturates	3.7g	7.3g	36.5%	20g	30g
mono-unsaturates	4.0g	7.9g	-	-	-
polyunsaturates	1.6g	3.2g	-	-	-
Fibre	2.3g	4.5g	18.8%	24g	24g
Salt	1.0g	2.0g	33.3%	6g	6g
of which sodium	0.4g	0.79g	32.9%	2.4g	2.4g

Nutrition Information — Guidelines

Low salt = 0.3 g or less per 100 g (or 0.1 g sodium)

NOTE: These figures are based on able-bodied guidelines and therefore adjustments may be required in the presence of a disability.

Junk food marketing to children campaign

Junk food influences children's choices.

Around 30 per cent of children in the UK are overweight or obese, and research shows that children are eating too much saturated fat and sugar. Obese children are more likely to become obese adults, which in turn increases their risk of developing a number of chronic health conditions, including cardiovascular disease, type 2 diabetes and some kinds of cancer. An unhealthy diet high in sugar also increases the risk of developing tooth decay. Children are also eating too much salt which increases the risk of high blood pressure, which in turn increases the risk of heart disease and stroke later in life.

Food and beverage producers aim to build long-term relationships between young consumers and their brands, and research shows that food promotions can influence children's behaviour in a number of ways including their preferences, purchase behaviour and consumption.

Children as young as 18 months can recognise brands and children as young as three have been shown to prefer branded, over identical unbranded food. Marketing therefore plays a significant role in influencing children's dietary choices. Sadly, the marketing of food and drinks to children is weighted heavily towards unhealthy foods, with very few advertisements promoting healthy options.

Children are also constantly exposed to junk food marketing: on TV, on radio, on the Internet, in e-mails, social media and text messages, at the cinema, in comics and magazines, in supermarkets, on food packaging, and for some even at school. Children should be protected from commercial interests that encourage them to eat foods that are high in saturated fat, salt and sugar. To improve their dietary health and life chances, they must be protected from the marketing of unhealthy food and drink. The recommendations in this article are also made by the National Institute for Health and Clinical Excellence (NICE) in its June 2010 report on the prevention of cardiovascular disease.

Marketers are exploiting loopholes in the regulation

TV: Regulation is already in place that prevents advertisements for unhealthy foods from being broadcast during or around programmes specifically made for children. However, the broadcast regulations are not strong enough because children also watch shows which most people consider to be family entertainment shows. The advertising industry, however, considers such programmes as 'adult' programming so they therefore fall outside of current regulations. Recent Ofcom statistics show that since the introduction of advertising restrictions, children's viewing habits have changed. They often watch television later in the evening, with their viewing during 'adult' commercial airtime now peaking during 8–9pm. A 9pm watershed on TV already exists to protect children from content which is unsuitable for a child audience. This should be extended to include unhealthy food and drink adverts to protect a vulnerable group.

Food manufacturers are using this to their advantage and advertising unhealthy products during some of the television programmes most popular with children, such as *The X-Factor* and *The Simpsons*, because these are not covered by the regulations. The case for stronger protection is reinforced by research which suggests that the current regulations are not working as children are exposed to the same number of advertisements for unhealthy food as before their introduction.

In addition, there is considerable popular support for action: a recent survey found that 65 per cent of adults agree that junk food adverts should be shown only after 9pm. The need for protective restrictions is recognised by the Broadcasting Authority of Ireland. In 2013 it

We asked young people whether they thought that junk food companies should be advertising their products directly to children. Here are a few of their answers:

'No, because if they are seeing food like this then they are more likely to want the unhealthy option rather than a healthier choice because they instantly think of the food they have most seen on the TV.' 16-year-old

'No, it's leading children to pressure their parents into buying them junk food.' 13-year-old

'Junk food adverts encourage children to buy unhealthy food and then they may become overweight.' 14-year-old

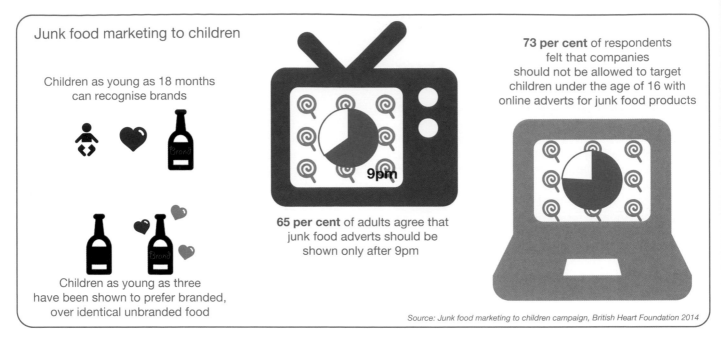

Junk food marketing to children

Children as young as 18 months can recognise brands

Children as young as three have been shown to prefer branded, over identical unbranded food

65 per cent of adults agree that junk food adverts should be shown only after 9pm

73 per cent of respondents felt that companies should not be allowed to target children under the age of 16 with online adverts for junk food products

Source: Junk food marketing to children campaign, British Heart Foundation 2014

introduced a ban on the television advertising for foods high in fat, sugar and salt before 6pm, a 25 per cent limit on the advertising sold for these foods after 6pm and rules to prevent the use of celebrities, characters, health claims or offers to promote unhealthy foods. It is now time for the UK Government and Ofcom to ensure that children in the UK are better protected.

Online and other non-broadcast media

The current self-regulatory system for non-broadcast advertising is weak and allows products which are outlawed from children's television to be marketed to children online. Websites for food and drinks almost exclusively promote products that are high in sugar and/or fat and/or salt, often using techniques which children will find difficult to identify as advertising – advergames, downloads and competitions, for example. Research shows that advergames, which are currently unregulated, are even more powerful than traditional advertising. This is because children are subconsciously targeted for longer periods of time, to engage with the brand or product through play rather than passive viewing. A BHF (British Heart Foundation) and Children's Food Campaign (CFC) report, *The 21st Century Gingerbread House,* demonstrates the exploitative nature of this kind of marketing. The CFC's follow up

report, *Through the Looking Glass*, demonstrates failings with the complaints procedure, which it finds weighted to the advantage of the food industry. Furthermore, in a BHF survey 73 per cent of respondents felt that companies should not be allowed to target children under the age of 16 with online adverts for junk food products.

Underpinning this problem are vague rules which do not differentiate between healthy and unhealthy foods, and fail to cover some key marketing techniques such as the use of brand characters. For example, the advertising code states that 'Marketing communications should not condone or encourage poor nutritional habits or an unhealthy lifestyle in children' – but what constitutes 'condoning and encouraging' or 'poor habits' is left open to interpretation.

The narrow remit of the advertising code also leaves a number of other marketing techniques – including sponsorship of events, placement at supermarket checkouts, and product-based marketing techniques such as packaging and food shape – completely unregulated, creating significant loopholes in the regulatory framework. Similarly, voluntary pledges such as the EU Pledge on responsible marketing are ineffective. The voluntary nature allows industry to set their own criteria for adhering to these

pledges creating further loopholes in the system in favour of industry's self-interest.

Action needed

1.   Move the responsibility for developing, monitoring, and evaluating advertising regulations to a body independent of the advertising industry.

2.   Amend regulations to prevent TV advertisements for unhealthy food and drinks before 9pm.

3.   Introduce consistent and effective regulations to protect under-16s across all forms of media. The new regulations should:

- Include all marketing techniques

- Distinguish between healthy and unhealthy products using a validated nutrient profiling model

- Establish a means of determining whether a product or promotion is targeting children.

⇨   The above information is reprinted with kind permission from the British Heart Foundation. Please visit www.bhf.org.uk for further information.

© British Heart Foundation 2014

Junk foods avoid ad ban by targeting children online

Campaign claims regulator failing to protect children from aggressive online marketing and child-friendly Internet games.

By Robert Booth

Advertising regulators have been accused of failing to protect children from aggressive online marketing by food companies using Internet games and advertising.

The Children's Food Campaign has called on ministers to introduce statutory regulation to close loopholes allowing ads that are banned from children's television to be shown on manufacturers' own child-friendly websites.

The campaign is supported by the British Medical Association, Diabetes UK and the National Obesity Forum. It wants limits on embedded online games such as the Haribo Super Mix Challenge, in which children are encouraged to collect sweets, or the Chewits Taste Adventure, where children have to find sweets hidden in British landmarks.

Singling out websites for Cadbury, Swizzels Matlow, Oreo and other brands, it said self-regulation by the advertising industry is failing and warned that the Internet has become an important battleground for children's diets, with evidence suggesting promotional games can subconsciously affect behaviour.

'Food companies continue to exploit loopholes and advertise junk foods to children online, even though stronger broadcasting regulations prevent such advertising on children's television,' said Malcolm Clark, co-ordinator of the campaign. 'The Advertising Standards Authority [ASA] is struggling to get to grips with its new role and is failing.'

The campaign group wants a crackdown on online claims about the nutritional value of snacks and greater control of child-friendly characters, such as the Sugar Puffs Honey Monster. The Soil Association, which promotes organic farming, and Organix, a brand of alternative children's snacks, are backing the calls for statutory regulation.

The ASA denied there was any need for a change in the law and said there was no evidence yet that any significant reform was needed, although it has launched a review of controls.

'After two years we can look back and ask what we could do better and it is being looked at seriously,' said Matt Wilson, a spokesman for the ASA. 'This industry has a 50-year history of making sure the rules remain relevant and appropriate. The advertising codes are robust around protecting children and the rules are based on the best available evidence about potential harms to children.'

The Children's Food Campaign filed complaints against 54 websites that promoted foods to children that were high in fat, salt or sugars, which it said 'failed to protect children from unhealthy food marketing'. The complaints were rejected outright by the ASA, which said they did not encourage irresponsible consumption. It added: 'We are not a social engineer and it is not our role to say whether a legally available product or service is good or bad.'

More detailed complaints about 19 websites, selected as the 'worst offenders', resulted in only two being partially upheld, two informally resolved and the rest rejected outright. A Pac-Man-style game that allowed players to guide the Honey Monster through a maze of Sugar Puffs was allowed because 'the consumption of Sugar Puffs had been represented in an abstract way', while a Swizzels game where the player could collect cola bottle sweets was ruled to have breached the code (see below).

The campaign group also challenged unrestricted access to TV-style adverts embedded in websites for Cadbury's Creme Eggs, Fanta orange drinks and Haribo sweets. No action was taken by the ASA, with the committee of advertising practice that draws up the code commenting there was 'an absence of evidence linking non-broadcast food advertising to dietary preferences... There is clearly a difference in likely impact between content appearing in a media that requires the user to access and content appearing unannounced during a TV schedule.'

A complaint about a Chewits website featuring Chewie the Chewitsaurus, a Kellogg's site with the Snap, Crackle and Pop characters and a Nestlé advert with Quicky the Nesquik rabbit were not investigated because rules to protect primary and pre-school children ban food and drink advertising from using celebrities and licensed characters, but not own-brand characters.

Food for thought: some of the complaints

Sugar Puffs

The 'Munching Monster' game on the website involved leading the Honey Monster around a maze eating cereal. The CFC said the game 'encourages excessive consumption of the product and poor nutritional habits'. Honey Monster Foods Ltd said no one had yet completed three levels of the game which is what it would take to consume 450 virtual puffs, enough for a 30 g bowl. They added a cup of coffee to the entry page to make it 'more adult-oriented'. The ASA said 'consumption of Sugar Puffs had been represented in an abstract way... players were unlikely to associate the Honey Monster's consumption with their own'.

Oreo

The CFC complained about a child-friendly advert for Oreo biscuits which showed a child consuming the product. The complaint was that the ad could not be shown on TV and it should be 'common sense for similar rules to apply, irrespective of the media'.

The ASA did not investigate and the Committee of Advertising Practice said it was 'not proportionate to mirror the TV scheduling rules in non-broadcast given the significant differences between TV and other media, not least the absence of evidence linking non-broadcast food advertising to dietary preferences'.

Swizzles

The Swizzles Town feature was aimed at pre-school and primary age children and promoted the company's sweets, CFC complained. Among several games it included Cola Capers where, the ASA concluded, 'the game's character could collect almost 100 cola bottle sweets. If the character was caught by the "angry parents" they would lose a life. We considered the game... condoned eating a large number of sweets while hiding from one's parents. [It] irresponsibly encouraged poor nutritional habits and an unhealthy lifestyle'. The company said the website contained information about products and did not encourage poor eating habits and was targeted at 'a family audience'.

29 April 2013

⇨ The above information is reprinted with kind permission from *The Guardian*. Please visit www.theguardian.com for further information.

Toddlers who eat the same meals as their parents are healthier

By Emilie King

Children who eat the same food as their parents have healthier diets, a recent study from the University of Edinburgh has found. Using a sample of over 2,000 four-year-olds in Scotland, Dr Valeria Skafida who carried out the research, found that youngsters who are fed the same food as the rest of the family eat more fruit and vegetables, less fatty and salty foods and snack less.

This had the greatest impact on a young child's health than any other factor – including eating together at mealtimes.

'Children are nutritionally better-off by eating the same food as their parents, and this holds independently of whether children eat meals together or not. Eating at the same time as the rest of the family or eating with parents, are not significantly associated with diet,' she said.

In the study, Dr Skafida pointed to the fact that food geared especially to children, either in the home or in restaurants, is not as nutritious as adult food.

'When children refuse to eat adult food during the family meal, it is a common coping strategy for parents to create separate and different child-friendly food alternatives often of inferior nutritional value to the family meal. This seems to be a widespread phenomenon, also reflected in child menus offered at restaurants which are typically of poorer nutritional value than adult equivalents,' she said.

Scotland has one of the worst obesity records in the developed world. One third of Scottish children are overweight or obese and these figures are on the rise, according to a 2012 Scottish Government report.

5 September 2013

⇨ The above information is reprinted with kind permission from Food Tank. Please visit www.foodtank.com for further information.

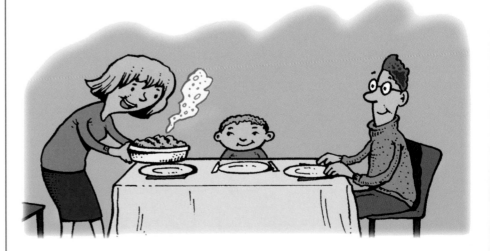

Healthy eating on a budget

You may not think it's possible to be frugal and follow a healthy diet at the same time. While some foods can be expensive, it doesn't necessarily mean they are the best.

You can still follow a healthy and balanced diet by shopping smart with our ten top tips.

1. Plan your meals

At the beginning of the week, take your time to make a grocery list of everything you need for your meals. This will help you buy only what you need and keep impulse purchases and overspending at bay.

2. Base your meals on starchy foods

These include bread, pasta, rice and potatoes, and are recommended to be the main energy source of your meals. Not only is it a tick in the box for healthy eating, these foods are easy on the purse strings too. Opt for wholemeal or brown versions where possible.

3. Keep your eyes peeled for special offers

Look out for cheaper or discounted food. If you see a product on offer that you use a lot, such as baked beans, canned tomatoes or tuna, stock up while you can. But

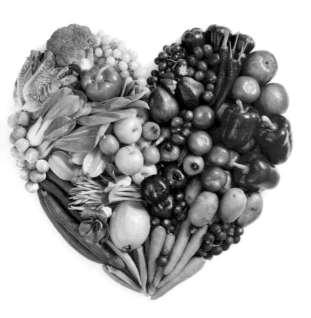

beware, unhealthy snacks are often the types of food on offer. Don't be tempted to buy cheap snacks, such as crisps or chocolate, to fill the cupboards.

4. Buy frozen fruit and vegetables

Frozen vegetables are often cheaper and will last a lot longer, helping to reduce what you waste. They still count towards your five-a-day, so stock up on the likes of frozen peas, sweetcorn and mixed berries. Frozen fruit and veg are great because they retain their vitamins and nutrients, which can be lost if they are fresh and not used for a while.

5. Try canned fish

You should aim to eat two portions of fish per week, one of which should be oily. Canned varieties of oily fish are often cheaper than fresh options, and have the added bonus of lasting much longer too. Go for ones in spring water to help keep your intake of salt down.

6. Bulk up your meals

Make your meals go further by adding canned tomatoes, beans and pulses, rice or pasta. These food products are all low-cost, as well as healthy additions. Add them to soups, stews and casseroles. Liquid-based meals are also a good option as they help you feel fuller for longer.

7. Watch what you drink

The best liquid to keep you hydrated is water, and it's free! Tap water in the UK is fine to drink and costs nothing more than a small addition to your water bill. Fizzy beverages and fruit juice drinks might be on offer, but they may not be healthy as they are full of sugar. Cross them off your shopping list to save some pennies.

If you enjoy an alcoholic drink, limit how much you have and when you have it. If you open a bottle of wine, try having just one glass with dinner, rather than finishing the bottle in one night. Not only will this benefit your health, it will make your beverage last for another time too.

8. Swap sugary cereals for porridge

Porridge oats are a great source of fibre. Not only is porridge cheap and simple to make, it's nutritious and will keep you full for the morning. A great way to help you to cut back on unhealthy mid-morning snacks and unnecessary spending.

9. Think about portion sizes

Many people often cook more than they need. Weigh out foods, such as pasta or rice, and if you do make too much, keep the leftovers for lunch or dinner. If you know you're not going to use it the next day, freeze it. Put it in an air-tight container or seal-lock bag and keep it in the freezer for a time when you need a quick meal.

10. Make staying in the new going out

Try to limit how much you eat out or how often you have a takeaway. Instead, cook at home, but make a night of it. Cook as a family, try something new, light some candles or invite friends over to join you. Pot luck meals, where everyone brings a dish, are a fun and money-saving way of eating together.

February 2014

⇨ The above information is reprinted with kind permission from Bupa. Please visit www.bupa.co.uk for further information.

FoodSwitch is an addictive app to help find healthier food

Working out what are the healthiest options in the supermarket can be a difficult job, especially when food labels are often designed to trick you into thinking they're healthier than they are. We asked one academic to road-test a new app that claims to help you clear up some of that confusion.

By Suzana Almoosawi, Research Associate at Newcastle University

Monday morning and here I am reaching my hand to a bowl full of my favourite granola. But wait, I have just downloaded this new app on my phone that helps me make healthier food choices by comparing the food labels of the foods I choose, versus alternatives with lower fat, saturated fat and salt content.

FoodSwitch is a free app that gives you advice to help you make healthier choices at your fingertips. The steps look easy: pick the product in the supermarket, scan the barcode, and receive a list of similar products that are lower in fat, saturated fat, and/or salt, *et voila*. It is then up to if you would like to share your options with relatives or friends who might be shopping for you or to create your own list of healthy alternatives so next time you are planning a shopping trip

you know where to find these new healthier foods.

The app was developed by academics and health campaigners and claims to be able to compare more than 80,000 food products from UK supermarkets using the traffic light system. And instead of you standing around flicking between one item in one hand and another in the other, they say, the app can do it for you.

Breakfast

Sounds all good but does it really work? To find out, I decided to test the app – starting with my cereal. I pick up my smartphone from the table and try to focus the camera on the barcode and snap, within a few microseconds I have a list of healthier options.

Tut tut, I should have realised it but my cereal has 25.4 g of fat, of which

2.8 g is saturated fat, probably from the pecan nuts and added oils. Naughty, but apparently I could still enjoy a bowl of granola every morning if I would go for the Tesco Finest Multi-grain Raspberry and Blueberries alternative; much lower in fat and only 3 g higher in sugars.

After that I get carried away. I decide to test the app on a few more cereals in the cupboard: Quaker Oat So Simple Apple & Blueberry, Weetabix Crunchy Bran – and others. Brilliant results, as I find myself with many alternatives that are almost half in saturated and contain three times less sugar.

Lunch

It's now lunchtime at work. I decide to test if my Innocent Strawberry and Banana Smoothie is so innocent after all. We all know that smoothies contain whole fruits and so unlike fruit juice they tend to retain a larger proportion of the goodness in fruit (though they can still be high in sugar). Using the app, I find there are more than six other more saintly versions of smoothies that I haven't thought of. Some are from the same brand and others are from other leading manufacturers. All of my new options had lower amounts of sugars and some were cheaper too. Not bad, seems like the app could help you remain trim while making sure your wallet remains less skinny.

Next up, my pot of Covent Garden vegetable soup with red split lentils, but this time I have made a good food choice – most of the alternatives come with a similar nutrient content, and occasionally with lower saturated fat content. Good to know the nutritionist in me has managed to pick up a good food choice.

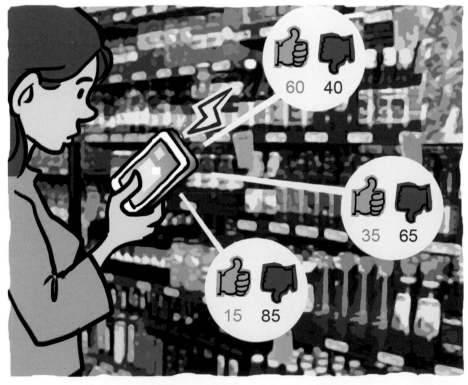

There's a danger the app could annoy those near you. My colleague is sitting next to me and is just about to have her little pot of Muller light Vanilla yoghurt at only 99 kcal per pot, but is it so light? I ask if she would mind me borrowing the pot and scanning the barcode to see if she could be getting something else for her lunch treat and not surprisingly there were a few options that could be in fact lighter.

Mind the gap

There were some gaps in the app's knowledge: it didn't contain nutrient information for most soups and in Marks and Spencer's Fuller Longer range of ready meals. Most, if not all, of the ready meals in Waitrose were not on the database. A lot of the organic brands (Duchy, Rachel's) were also missing.

The developers have an answer to this: crowdsourcing. By taking three photos of a missing item and uploading it to the app they say it will be added to the system and become available to all users.

Occasionally, the app misses the point and just like a wise dietitian, it can find it challenging to choose between which is better: lower fat or lower salt, for example. This happened especially with products like yoghurts and some ready meals, and when it got slightly tricky in terms of choosing what was right for me.

Using FoodSwitch in conjunction with another app that allowed me to estimate my daily nutrient intake would also have made it easier to make an overall informed choice about my daily diet.

There are a number of these on the market including MyFitnessPal, which has one of the largest food databases in a diet tracker, and CRON-O-Meter, which is free and simple to use. Using one of these along with FoodSwitch would give you the full picture.

11 April 2014

⇨ The above information is reprinted with kind permission from The Conversation. Please visit www.theconversation.com for further information.

How do I know if a processed food is high in fat, saturated fat, sugar or salt?

There are guidelines to tell you if a food is high or low in fat, saturated fat, salt or sugar. These are:

Total fat

High: more than 17.5 g of fat per 100 g

Low: 3 g of fat or less per 100 g

Saturated fat

High: more than 5 g of saturated fat per 100 g

Low: 1.5 g of saturated fat or less per 100 g

Sugars

High: more than 22.5 g of total sugars per 100 g

Low: 5 g of total sugars or less per 100 g

Salt

High: more than 1.5 g of salt per 100 g (or 0.6 g sodium)

Low: 0.3 g of salt or less per 100 g (or 0.1 g sodium)

For example, if you are trying to cut down on saturated fat, try to limit the amount of foods you eat that have more than 5 g of saturated fat per 100 g.

If the processed food you want to buy has a nutrition label that uses colour-coding, you will often find a mixture of red, amber and green. So, when you're choosing between similar products, try to go for more greens and ambers, and fewer reds, if you want to make a healthier choice.

However, even healthier ready meals may be higher in fat and other additives than a homemade equivalent. That's not to say that homemade foods can't also be high in calories, fat, salt and sugar, but if you make the meal yourself, you'll have a much better idea of what's gone into it. You could even save yourself some money, too.

1 June 2014

⇨ **The above information is reprinted with kind permission from NHS Choices. Please visit www.nhs.uk for further information.**

The draft School Food Standards

Eating in school should be a pleasurable experience, a time spent sharing good food with peers and teachers.

These standards are intended to ensure that children get the nutrition they need across the whole school day. It is just as important to cook food that looks good and tastes good; to talk to children about what is on offer and recommend dishes; to reduce queuing; and to serve the food in a pleasant environment where they can eat with their friends.

As a general principle, it is important to provide a wide range of foods across the week. Variety is key – whether it is different fruits, vegetables, grains, pulses or types of meat and fish. Wherever possible, foods should be prepared in the school's own kitchen from fresh, locally sourced ingredients.

* This Standard applies across the whole school day, including breakfasts, morning breaks, tuck shops, and after school clubs

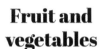

Fruit and vegetables

One or more portions of vegetables as an accompaniment every day.

One or more portions of fruit every day. A dessert containing at least 50% fruit two or more times each week.

At least three different fruits and three different vegetables each week.

Foods high in fat, sugar and salt

No more than two portions of food that has been deep-fried, batter-coated, or breadcrumb-coated each week.*

No more than two portions of food which include pastry each week.*

No snacks, except nuts, seeds, vegetables and fruit with no added salt, sugar or fat.*

Savoury crackers or breadsticks can be served at lunch with fruit or vegetables or dairy food.

No confectionery, chocolate or chocolate-coated products.*

Desserts, cakes and biscuits are allowed only at lunchtime. They must not contain any confectionery as ingredients.

Salt must not be available to add to food after it has been cooked.*

Any condiments limited to sachets or portions of no more than 10g or one teaspoonful.*

Milk and dairy

A portion of food from this group every day.

Low fat milk available for drinking every day.

Meat, fish, eggs, beans

and other non-dairy sources of protein

A portion of food from this group every day.

A portion of meat or poultry on three or more days each week.

Oily fish once or more every three weeks.

A portion of non-dairy sources of protein available three or more days each week for vegetarians.

A meat or poultry product (manufactured or homemade and meeting the legal requirements no more than once each week in primary schools and twice each week in secondary schools.*

Food provided outside lunch

• Fruit and/or vegetables available in all school food outlets.

• No savoury crackers and breadsticks.

• No cakes, biscuits, pastries or desserts (except yoghurt).

Starchy food

One or more wholegrain varieties of starchy food each week.

One or more portions of food from this group every day.

Three or more different starchy foods each week.

Starchy food cooked in fat or oil no more than two days each week.*

Bread (with no added fat or oil) must be available every day.

Healthier drinks*

Free, fresh drinking water at all times.

The only drinks permitted are:

• Plain water (still or carbonated); low fat milk or lactose reduced milk;

• Fruit or vegetable juice; (max 150 mls);

• Plain soya, rice or oat drinks enriched with calcium; plain fermented milk (e.g. yoghurt) drinks;

• Unsweetened combinations of fruit or vegetable juice with plain water (still or carbonated);

• Combinations of fruit juice and low fat milk or plain low fat yoghurt, plain soya, rice or oat drinks enriched with calcium; cocoa and low fat milk; flavoured low fat milk;

• Tea, coffee, hot chocolate.

Combination drinks are limited to a portion size of 330ml. They may contain added vitamins or minerals, but no more than 5% added sugars or honey or 150ml of fruit content. Fruit juice combination drinks must be at least 45% fruit juice.

Source: Revised standards for food in schools, Department of Education, 17 June 2014. © Crown copyright 2014

Tesco to educate every child about food and where it comes from

Every primary school in the UK will be given the chance to learn more about food and where it comes from as part of a major new food education programme launched today.

Farm to Fork, the first initiative from The Tesco Eat Happy Project, is backed by supporters including Diabetes UK, the Children's Food Trust and the NFU. From the end of February kids will be able to go on educational Farm to Fork Trails in factories, on farms and in supermarkets, for practical demonstrations of where food comes from and how it is made.

The ambition is to take one million of the five million primary school children in the UK on the Farm to Fork Trails in the project's first year.

Through technology, classes will also have the opportunity to talk to food suppliers across the world, for example banana growers in Costa Rica, through Google+ hangouts and live video chats, using Google's Connected Classrooms. Tesco is also partnering with Sorted Food, Europe's largest social media cooking channel to engage children with content that makes cooking fun and accessible.

The Tesco Eat Happy Project is a commitment to improving children's relationship with food and it forms part of the company's wider ambition to help and encourage all of its customers and colleagues to lead healthier and more active lives. With eating habits starting in early childhood, Tesco aims to help primary school children learn and have a healthier relationship with food.

The project launches as new research from the Future Foundation reveals that even though 90 per cent of kids say they know which foods are healthy, fewer than ten per cent achieve their five-a-day target. More than half (52 per cent) believe potatoes count towards the total, and one in ten (ten per cent) also count carrot cake.

The Future Foundation report highlights British parents' concerns about their kids' relationship with food: two-thirds believe children eat much more convenience food than they did and an astounding 80 per cent say their kids are less healthy than they themselves used to be as kids. Half of parents fear the impact of their children's diet on long-term health.

In light of these findings, Tesco is pledging £15 million to the Eat Happy Project in the first year alone.

Farm to Fork is the first initiative of The Tesco Eat Happy Project. Developed in close working with teachers and in line with the curriculum, Farm to Fork will involve:

⇨ Specially trained colleagues in more than 700 Tesco stores across the UK teaching kids about different foods and giving practical demonstrations, for example baking bread, tasting new fruits and vegetables and learning all about fish.

⇨ Food suppliers across the country opening their farms and factories to teach kids how, for example, milk is produced, where eggs come from and how lettuce grows.

⇨ Tesco partnering with Sorted Food, Europe's largest social media cooking channel. The Sorted team will help to engage people with content that makes cooking social, fun and accessible.

⇨ An innovative new partnership with Google's Connected Classrooms, through which Tesco will become the first company in the UK to offer educational 'virtual field trips' for primary schools to talk to producers and Tesco colleagues around the world.

⇨ A dedicated website with lesson plans, recipes and 'how to' videos for children, parents and teachers.

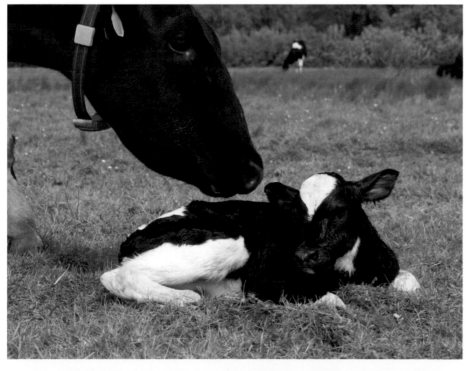

The Farm to Fork Trails and Connected Classrooms will be open to every primary school in the UK.

Tesco UK Managing Director, Chris Bush, said:

'We know parents are concerned that kids don't always understand how food is made and where it comes from, which is important to developing a strong positive lifelong relationship with food. Working closely with teachers, our suppliers and a number of partners including the Children's Food Trust, we want to help make the relationship primary school kids have with food better, and that's the aim of the Eat Happy Project. It's part of our ambition to help all of our customers and colleagues lead healthier lives and just one of the ways we are using our scale to help communities across the UK.'

The second phase of The Tesco Eat Happy Project, to launch later in the year, will involve cookery courses for kids in stores, working with the Children's Food Trust.

Peter Kendall, President of the NFU, said:

'The NFU welcomes this initiative which encourages children to learn more about where their food comes from and the important role British farming has in producing traceable and sustainable food. Children of today will become the food-buyers of the future and we hope this scheme helps to increase loyalty and support for British farmers and the high-quality food we produce.'

Pete Mountstephen, Chair of the Primary Heads Association, said:

'The key to reconnecting kids' knowledge of food to what they eat is getting them excited, at a young age, about where their favourite food comes from and how it gets to their plate. Schoolchildren across the UK definitely have the appetite to learn, engage and understand more about the provenance of their favourite meals and in particular discover and explore the farms and other suppliers of that food.

'I'm hugely excited about the Farm to Fork initiative and the aims of

The Tesco Eat Happy Project and I have no doubt the UK's primary schoolchildren will thoroughly enjoy their experiences on the Farm to Fork Trails.'

Simon O'Neill, Diabetes UK's Director of Health Intelligence, said:

'The Tesco Eat Happy Project is a great initiative that will help children understand the importance of eating a healthy balanced diet. The best way to reduce the risk of developing type 2 diabetes in the future – whatever age you are – is to maintain a healthy weight by eating a healthy, balanced diet and by being regularly physically active. Making sensible food choices and adapting your eating habits can also help people with diabetes to better manage their condition and avoid complications.'

Carmel McConnell, Founder of children's education and health charity, Magic Breakfast, said:

'Most children need active encouragement to go outside their favourite food habits, to try different types of food, in the correct proportions, in order to have a healthy and well-balanced diet. However many families don't have the money, or time, or food awareness to be able to do this successfully, which can mean children miss out on vital nutrients, as well as the chance to discover new flavours and recipes. So, in trying to broaden the food horizons of a million primary school children, The Tesco Eat Happy Project looks like a welcome and ambitious new approach to children's food education and I am pleased to be able to give my support to a great scheme encouraging healthier family eating.'

Marvin Chow, Global Marketing Director for Google+, said:

'We're delighted to work with Tesco on their food education programme through Google+ Connected Classrooms to bring their virtual field trips to classrooms in the UK and globally via Google+ Hangouts. It's great to see a brand use Google+ technology to educate children on where food comes from,

helping them develop a healthier relationship with it.'

Jamie Spafford, Sorted Food, said:

'Sorted's mission has always been to get young people into the kitchen cooking up great food. The Eat Happy Project seems like a great way to get that message out to more people, and helps to kick start the health of the next generation.'

Linda Cregan, Chief Executive of the Children's Food Trust said:

'Everyone at the Children's Food Trust is looking forward to working with Tesco on this exciting new project. Improving the diets of our children should be a priority for all of us. Parents, schools and food retailers and manufacturers all have a responsibility to make sure our children are eating healthy, nutritious food. If our children grow up with an understanding and interest in both cooking and eating healthy food they have the best opportunity to reach their full potential.

'Being overweight or obese from an early age puts our children at a massive disadvantage from the word go and we can all support parents in safeguarding their children's health.

'As the country's biggest supermarket chain it is fantastic Tesco are taking the initiative to make this change. Encouraging the nation to improve its diet is a huge challenge and we need companies like Tesco to get involved if we are going to make a change. With their influence, resources and reach we're sure they can make a big difference to our children's diet.'

27 January 2014

⇨ The above information is reprinted with kind permission from Farming News. Please visit www.farming.co.uk for further information.

We would urge the Scottish Government to state clearly that there is no place for Tesco to teach food education in Scottish schools

By Mike Small

We're delighted to support the announcement of free school meals for all schoolchildren in Scotland from primary one to three from next January. This is a key next step in the food revolution – but one that needs to be matched with local procurement, use of fresh seasonal ingredients and high nutritional standards to maximise its impact. The move will affect 165,000 youngsters, and is claimed will boost health and educational attainment. It will also save families £330 a year for each child. The £114 million package will provide free school meals to pupils in P1 to P3 and extend free nursery provision to thousands more two-year-olds. The extra childcare will be targeted at the most deprived pupils.

Congratulations to the coalition of groups who won the argument and received a victory for social justice: Children in Scotland, Children 1ST, Save the Children, One Parent Families Scotland, the Child Poverty Action Group, the Educational Institute of Scotland (EIS), STUC, UNISON, Church of Scotland, Shelter Scotland and the Poverty Alliance.

Anti-poverty campaigners, children's organisations, trade unions and faith groups have long argued that the most effective way of ensuring all children, but particularly those in poverty, receive a healthy school lunch is to move toward a universal, non-means tested approach to the provision of healthy lunches in the middle of the school day (see http://www.cpag.org.uk/scotland/school-meals).

Graeme Brown, Director of Shelter Scotland has said:

'At a time when the pressure on household budgets is forcing many families to make hard choices and cut back on essentials, this move by the Scottish Government is very much welcomed by Shelter Scotland. Coming against the backdrop of further cuts in welfare – with more drastic reductions threatened yesterday by Chancellor George Osborne – free school meals for pupils in P1 to P3 is a direct and proven way of supporting, in particular, families on low or limited incomes, and helping all schoolchildren in Scotland enjoy a better, healthier start to their primary education.'

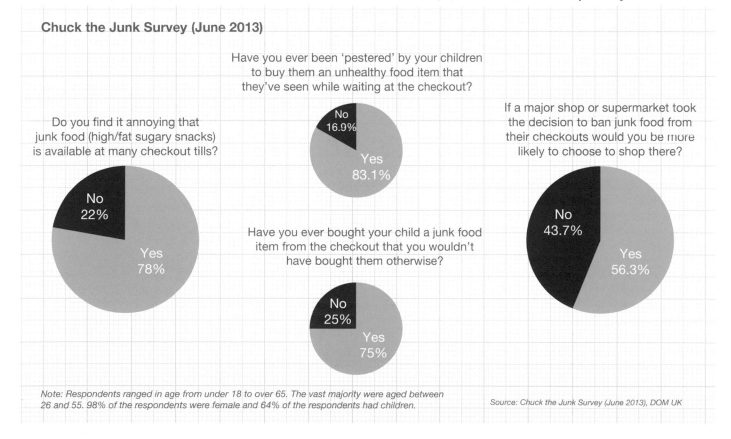

Chuck the Junk Survey (June 2013)

Do you find it annoying that junk food (high/fat sugary snacks) is available at many checkout tills?
No 22%
Yes 78%

Have you ever been 'pestered' by your children to buy them an unhealthy food item that they've seen while waiting at the checkout?
No 16.9%
Yes 83.1%

Have you ever bought your child a junk food item from the checkout that you wouldn't have bought them otherwise?
No 25%
Yes 75%

If a major shop or supermarket took the decision to ban junk food from their checkouts would you be more likely to choose to shop there?
No 43.7%
Yes 56.3%

Note: Respondents ranged in age from under 18 to over 65. The vast majority were aged between 26 and 55. 98% of the respondents were female and 64% of the respondents had children.

Source: Chuck the Junk Survey (June 2013), DOM UK

The key to success is not just making meals free but desirable and high quality, opening the door to a new menu of aspiration of food for life. Luckily there's evidence it will do just that. Recent research from the Institute for Social and Economic Research at the University of Essex also analysed the wider impact of the Scottish Government's free school meal pilots. The paper 'attributes the rise in take-up of FSMs by those always entitled to a positive peer effect: FSM-registered individuals became more likely to participate because a greater proportion of other students in the school were doing so... The magnitude of the effect is such that in a typical school a ten percentage point rise in peer-group take-up would reduce non-participation (i.e. non-take up by those already entitled) by almost a quarter.'

John Dickie, head of the Child Poverty Action Group (CPAG) defended specifically the universal nature of these changes, saying:

'A universal approach to healthy free school lunches provides a huge boost to children and parents at a time when they are under increasing pressure from tax credit and benefit cuts, soaring food and energy prices and stagnating wages. Current means-testing means too many of our worst-off children are not receiving a free school meal and parents too often struggle to meet the extra costs of lunches as they move back into work or increase their hours when their children start school. What's more, a universal approach ensures that all our children, whatever their home circumstances, gain the health and education benefits of a healthy lunch in the middle of the school day.'

The Fife Diet welcome this move but we also support the comments from Alison Johnston, Green MSP who added: 'Rolling out free school meals is a welcome, common sense move but ministers must also address what is being served up to our children. Our councils need support to make buying choices which have positive impacts for

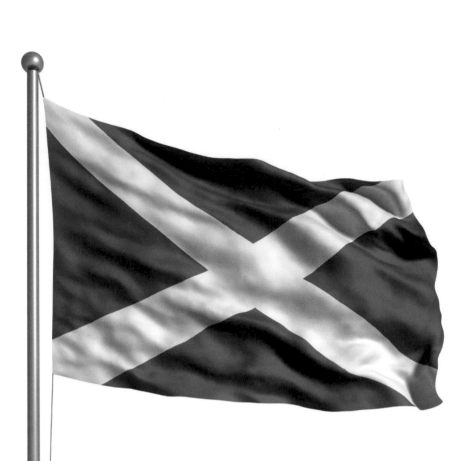

local farmers and producers. I will continue to put pressure on ministers so that they do not waste this golden opportunity.'

While Laura Stewart, Director of the Soil Association has stated:

Today's announcement of universal free school meals for P1-P3 pupils in Scotland is a welcome investment in our children's health and well-being. It has the potential to have a far-reaching effect on Scotland's food culture, in schools and beyond the school gates. It is vital, however, that cooks, teachers, parents and children are reassured that free school meals will be high quality, sustainable and tasty. We need to grasp this opportunity and build on some of the great work already happening in our schools. We must invest, not just in free school meals, but in skilled cooks creating fresh, healthy, sustainable and trustworthy meals too, delivered in a pleasant environment and supporting good eating habits.'

The universal approach has not only been shown to increase take up of healthy lunches and relief to family budgets but also to impact positively on children's learning experience. Evaluation of a free school meals pilot for primary school children over two years in Hull found a 'significant impact in all areas of children's schooling... behaviour, social relationships, health and learning', whilst more recent evaluation of the provision of free school meals to all primary pupils in Durham and Newham found that 'offering free school meals to all primary school pupils increased attainment in disadvantaged areas'.

30 January 2014

⇨ The above information is reprinted with kind permission from Fife Diet. Please visit www.fifediet.co.uk for further information.

© Fife Diet 2014

The eatwell plate

If you want to get the balance of your diet right, use the eatwell plate.

The eatwell plate makes healthy eating easier to understand by showing the types and proportions of foods we need to have a healthy and well-balanced diet.

The eatwell plate shows how much of what you eat should come from each food group. This includes everything you eat during the day, including snacks.

So, try to eat:

⇨ plenty of fruit and vegetables

⇨ plenty of bread, rice, potatoes, pasta and other starchy foods – choose wholegrain varieties whenever you can

⇨ some milk and dairy foods

⇨ some meat, fish, eggs, beans and other non-dairy sources of protein

⇨ just a small amount of foods and drinks high in fat and/or sugar.

Look at the eatwell plate to see how much of your food should come from each food group. You don't need to get the balance right at every meal. But try to get it right over time such as a whole day or week.

Try to choose options that are lower in fat, salt and sugar when you can.

⇨ The above information is reprinted with kind permission from the Food Standards Agency. Please visit www.eatwell.gov.uk for further information.

The eatwell plate

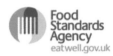

Use the eatwell plate to help you get the balance right. It shows how much of what you eat should come from each food group.

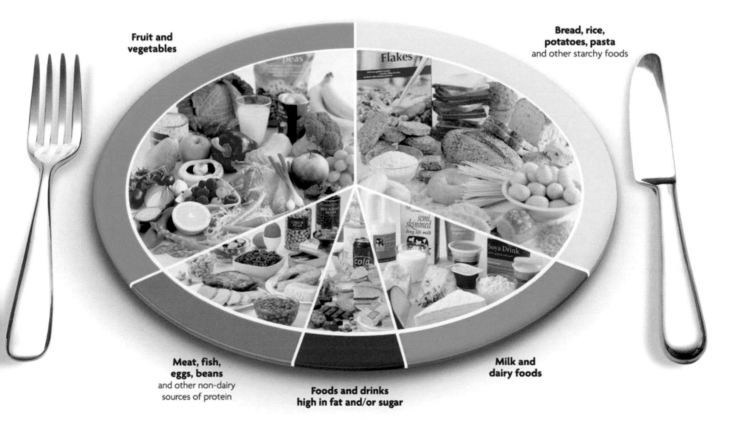

Key facts

- In mid-Victorian England obesity was virtually unknown except in the numerically small upper-middle and upper classes. (page 1)

- The average UK family is wasting nearly £60 a month by throwing away almost an entire meal a day. (page 2)

- The top three foods being thrown away uneaten in British homes are bread, potatoes and milk. The equivalent of 24 million slices of bread, 5.8 million potatoes and 5.9 million glasses of milk are being wasted daily. (page 2)

- [Oxfam] estimate that over 500,000 people are now reliant on food aid – the use of food banks and receipt of food parcels – and this number is likely to escalate further over the coming months. (page 3)

- Research conducted by the British Nutrition Foundation (BNF) among over 27,500 children across the UK, shows that nearly a third (29 per cent) of primary school children think that cheese comes from plants, one in ten secondary school children believe that tomatoes grow under the ground, and nearly one in five (18 per cent) primary school children say that fish fingers come from chicken. (page 5)

- 67 per cent of primary school children and 81 per cent of secondary school pupils reported eating four or less portions of fruit and vegetables daily, while two in every five children at secondary school don't think that frozen fruit and vegetables count towards their five a day. (page 5)

- 17 per cent of primary school children and 19 per cent of secondary school children cook at home either every day or once a week. However, nine per cent of children at primary school and 11 per cent of children at secondary school never cook at home. (page 5)

- The Foresight report (2007) concluded that half the UK population could be obese by 2050 at a cost of £50 billion per year. However, upward trends in obesity levels suggest these conclusions could be optimistic and could be exceeded by 2050. (page 6)

- [According to the 2013 report from the UN Food and Agriculture Organisation], the UK has the highest level of obesity in Western Europe, ahead of countries such as France, Germany, Spain and Sweden. (page 8)

- In England, 24.8% of adults are obese and 61.7% are either overweight or obese, according to the Health and Social Care Information Centre. (page 8)

- Energy drinks can contain high levels of caffeine, usually about 80 milligrams (mg) of caffeine in a small 250 ml can – the same as three cans of cola or a mug of instant coffee. (page 10)

- The UK sweetener sector is valued at £60 million, and more than a quarter of British households buy artificial sweeteners. (page 11)

- A new study, published in *BMJ Open*, suggests that a 15% drop in daily salt intake in England between 2003 and 2011 led to 42% less stroke deaths and a 40% drop in deaths from coronary heart disease. (page 12)

- Cutting the amount of saturated fat we eat by just 15 per cent could prevent around 2,600 premature deaths every year from conditions such as cardiovascular disease, heart disease and stroke. (page 13)

- In the UK, the Department of Health suggests that no more than 35% of total calories should come from fat. (page 14)

- Nutrition experts worldwide recommend that adults and children above the age of two obtain at least 50% of their daily calories from a variety of carbohydrate sources. (page 17)

- Around 30 per cent of children in the UK are overweight or obese, and research shows that children are eating too much saturated fat and sugar. (page 27)

- Children as young as 18 months can recognise brands and children as young as three have been shown to prefer branded, over identical unbranded food. (page 27)

- Children who eat the same food as their parents have healthier diets, a recent study from the University of Edinburgh has found. (page 30)

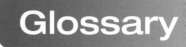

Glossary

Additives

Additives are ingredients used in the preparation of processed foods. Some of these are extracted from naturally occurring materials, others are manufactured chemicals. They may be added to food to stop it going bad (preservatives), improve its appearance (for example by changing its colour) or to enhance its flavour. Other types of additives include thickeners, sweeteners, emulsifiers and anti-caking agents, and there are many more.

Body Mass Index (BMI)

An individual's body mass index is calculated by applying a formula to their weight and height to determine if they are within a healthy weight range. A healthy individual has a BMI of between 20 and 25. Someone with a BMI of 30 or above would be classed as obese.

Diet

The variety of food and drink that someone eats on a regular basis. The phrase 'on a diet' is also often used to refer to a period of controlling what one eats while trying to lose weight.

Eatwell plate

The eatwell plate shows the different types of food we need to eat – and in what proportions – to have a well-balanced and healthy diet. Based on the eatwell plate, people should try to eat: plenty of fruit and vegetables; plenty of potatoes, bread, rice, pasta and other starchy foods; some milk and dairy foods; some meat, fish, eggs, beans and other non-dairy sources of protein; and just a small amount of foods and drinks that are high in fat or sugar.

Fat

Fat is an essential part of our diet. Our bodies require small amounts of 'good fat' to function and help prevent disease. However, too much fat, especially of the wrong type of fat, can cause serious health problems such as obesity, higher blood pressure and cholesterol levels, which in turn lead to a greater risk of heart disease. The two main types of fat are saturated and unsaturated. Unsaturated fats (e.g. found in oily fish) are generally considered better for us than saturated fats (such as dairy products, like cheese).

Fibre

Dietary fibre (sometimes called 'roughage') is the part of fruit, vegetables and wholefoods which cannot be digested by the body. It aids digestion by giving the gut bulk to squeeze against in order to move food through the digestive system. There are two types of fibre: soluble and insoluble.

Food poverty

When people struggle to afford food. The UK has seen an increase in the use of food banks and food parcels. The Trussel Trust food bank network provided over 350,000 people in the UK with food parcels in 2012-2013 – more than double the year before.

Junk food

'Junk' food is a widely-used term for unhealthy and fatty food with little nutritional value. It is usually associated with 'fast' or takeaway food.

Malnutrition

Malnutrition essentially means 'poor nutrition'. There are two types of malnutrition: undernutrition (when a person's diet is lacking in nutrients and sustenance they need) and overnutrition (when a person's diet is getting far too many nutrients for the body to cope with). Malnutrition can affect anybody, although it tends to be more common in developing countries where there are shortages of food.

Nutrition

The provision of materials needed by the body for growth, maintenance and sustaining life. Commonly when people talk about nutrition, they are referring to the healthy and balanced diet we all need to eat in order for the body to function properly.

Obesity

When someone is overweight to the extent that their BMI is 30 or above, they are classed as obese. Obesity is increasing in the UK and is associated with a number of health problems, including heart disease and diabetes.

Protein

Proteins are chains of amino acids that allow the body to build and repair body tissue. Protein is found in dairy foods, meat, fish and soya beans.

Starch

Starch is a complex carbohydrate found in potatoes, rice, corn, wheat and other foods. It is made up of glucose and allows animals and plants to store energy as fat.

Sugar

Sugar is a carbohydrate that is a naturally-occurring nutrient that makes food taste sweet. There are a number of different sugars: glucose and fructose are found in fruit and vegetables; milk sugar is known as lactose; maltose (malt sugar) is found in malted drinks and beer; and sucrose comes from sugar cane or beet and is often referred to as 'table' or 'added' sugar. It also occurs naturally in some fruit and vegetables.

Sweeteners

Artificial sweeteners are a low-calorie/calorie-free chemical substances used instead of sugar. They are found in thousands of products, such as drinks, desserts, ready meals and even toothpaste. There is much debate on the potential toxic side effects of consuming sweeteners.

Traffic light labelling

A new food labelling system, implemented by large food manufacturers and supermarkets to provide clear nutritional information to their consumers. Red, amber and green labels are used on food packaging to indicate how healthy that food is considered, with a green label indicating a very healthy food and red indicating a food that is high in salt, sugar or fats and which should therefore be enjoyed only in moderation.

Vitamins

Organic compounds that are essential to the body, but only in very small quantities. Most of the vitamins and minerals we need are provided through a balanced diet: however, some people choose to take additional vitamin supplements.

Assignments

Brainstorming

⇨ In small groups, discuss what you know about food and diet. Consider the following points:

- What is the eatwell plate?

- What is food poverty?

- What is food waste? How can it be avoided?

- What is Body Mass Index (BMI) and how is it used to measure whether someone is a healthy weight? Is it a useful tool? Can you think of any problems with the way BMI is calculated?

Research

⇨ How many cookery and food-related programmes are shown on television in the course of a week? Do any of these programmes explore healthy eating? Over the course of a week, make a note of all the food-related programmes you come across. Share your findings with your class and discuss why you think cooking/food programmes are popular, and whether they encourage or discourage healthy eating.

⇨ How much food do you throw away? Over the course of two weeks, keep track of how much food waste your household produces. How could this food waste have been avoided? Write a report analysing your findings and include suggestions for how you might reduce your household food waste in future.

⇨ In recent years, the nutritional value of school dinners has come under scrutiny. Carry out your own research into the issue of school meals, looking at campaigns such as Jamie Oliver's 'Feed Me Better' project. How healthy are the meals served in your own school canteen? Do you think they could be improved? Make some notes and feedback to your class.

⇨ How much sugar do you eat? Over the course of one day, make a note of how much sugar is contained in everything you eat. Are you adhering to government guidelines? Are you surprised by the volume of sugar in certain foods? Make some notes and discuss with your class.

Design

⇨ Design a leaflet explaining food poverty in Britain. You should describe what food banks and food parcels are. You might also want to include details about organisations people can turn to if they are experiencing difficulties, such as information about the Trussell Trust.

⇨ Create a poster that clearly explains the traffic light colour-coded food labels.

⇨ Create your own cookbook which includes recipes on the theme of 'eating healthy on a budget'. Think of a name for your cookbook and include at least three original recipes.

⇨ Design an informative leaflet that details the signs and symptoms of malnutrition. You may wish to include information about what treatment there is for malnutrition. Read *Malnutrition* on pages 4-5 and see the article in full at http://www.nutritionist-resource.org.uk/articles/malnutrition.html.

⇨ Choose one of the articles from this book and create your own illustration that highlights the key themes of the text.

Oral

⇨ With a partner, role-play a radio interview on the topic of 'greener food'. The interviewee, a campaigner for an environmental charity, should give advice on how our food affects the environment, how we can purchase climate-friendly and sustainable food and how we can produce less waste.

⇨ Choose one of the illustrations from this book and, with a partner, discuss what you think the artist was trying to portray.

⇨ Choose a country outside of Europe and research their relationship with food. How does it differ from the situation in the UK? What foods are traditionally eaten? Create a PowerPoint presentation that compares and contrasts your chosen country's food and diet with those of the UK.

⇨ Imagine that you have been asked to run a parents' evening at your school. The theme of the evening is 'healthy eating' and its aim is to educate and inform parents about the nutritional value of food. In groups, create a ten-minute presentation that will introduce parents to the eatwell plate and explore the theme of healthy eating. Remember that your presentation should be engaging, but not patronising.

Reading/writing

⇨ Read *Cheese comes from plants and fish fingers are made of chicken* on page 5 and create a lesson plan that would teach five-year-old children about where their food comes from.

⇨ Read *How has what we eat changed?* on pages 1-2. Write a short essay exploring how food and diet has changed over time. You might want to look at the ways in which food and diet have been affected by modern conveniences.

⇨ Jack Monroe is an active campaigner about the politics of food banks. She has a blog called A Girl Called Jack (www.agirlcalledjack.com) which debates the causes of food bank use and hunger in Britain, as well as sharing recipes for eating well on a budget. Visit Jack's site and choose a recipe to test. Write a blog entry exploring your thoughts about the recipe (you could also include some pictures of your finished dish!).

⇨ Write a letter to your headteacher explaining why you believe it is important for students to be taught about diet and nutrition at school.

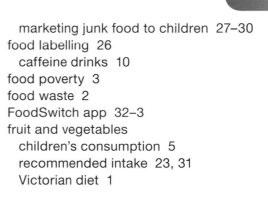

Action on Sugar campaign group 20
additives in food 10
alcohol 25
artificial sweeteners 11

balanced meals 25, 39
benefit system changes and food poverty 3
blood pressure effects of salt 12
BMI (body mass index) 14–15
breakfast 25
    children not eating 5
    healthy eating choices 31, 32

caffeine drinks 10, 24
calcium-rich foods 23–4
calorie intake 23
    Victorian diet 1
Change4Life 6
children
    behavioural effects of food additives 10
    eating same meals as parents 30
    and healthy eating 5
    and junk food marketing 27–30
    overweight 8, 20
    Tesco food education programme 35–6
    see also schools
Children's Food Campaign 29
cholesterol 15–16
Chunk the Junk survey 37
cooking experience, children 5
Cuba, reversing obesity problem 9

depression and malnutrition 4
deprivation and obesity 8
diet
    healthy see healthy eating
    Victorian era 1–2
diet-related malnutrition 5
doctors and obesity management 6–7

Eat Happy Project, Tesco 35–6
eatwell plate 25, 39
education about food and nutrition 5
    Tesco programme 35–6
    see also schools
essential fatty acids 14

family meals encouraging healthy eating 30
Farm to Fork programme, Tesco 35–6
fat 14–16
fibre 23
fish
    children's consumption of 5
    recommended intake 24, 31
fluid intake 7, 25, 31
food additives 10
food industry
    encouraging healthy choices 6, 13–14

marketing junk food to children 27–30
food labelling 26
    caffeine drinks 10
food poverty 3
food waste 2
FoodSwitch app 32–3
fruit and vegetables
    children's consumption 5
    recommended intake 23, 31
    Victorian diet 1

Government policy on obesity 6–7, 9
GPs and obesity management 6–7

health effects
    of fat 14, 15–16, 22
    of obesity 9, 20
    of salt 12
    of sugar 18–19, 21
health problems and malnutrition 4
healthy eating
    on a budget 31
    FoodSwitch app 32–3
    guidelines 23–5, 39
    schools 6, 34
Healthy Lives, Healthy People 9
high caffeine content drinks 10
hydration 7, 25, 31
hydrogenated (trans) fat 15

illness and malnutrition 4
ingredients lists on labels 26
    sugars 17
insulin 21
Internet games and junk food advertising 28, 29–30

junk food
    marketing to children 27–30
    survey 37

labelling of food 26
    caffeine drinks 10
lifestyle and obesity 8
low cost healthy eating 31

malnutrition 4
marketing of junk food to children 27–30
medical conditions and malnutrition 4
mental health problems and malnutrition 4
monounsaturated fat 15

nutrition labels 26, 33
nutritional supplements and malnutrition 4

obesity 6–7, 8–9
 in children 8, 20
 health consequences 9, 20
obesogenic environments 8
online advertising of junk food 28, 29–30
Oreo, complaints about marketing 30
overnutrition 4

physical activity and obesity 8
physical education, government guidelines 6
polyols 11
polyunsaturated fat 15
poverty and food aid 3
processed foods 24, 33
protein 24

Responsibility Deal 6
 Saturated Fat Reduction Pledge 13-14

salt consumption
 cutting down 24
 health effects 12
 Victorians 2
saturated fat 15
 reduction 13–14, 24
School Food Standards 34
schools
 healthy living guidelines 6
 School Food Standards 34
 school meals 6, 37–8
 Tesco food education programme 35–6

Scotland, free school meals 37–8
social factors
 and malnutrition 4
 and obesity 8
soft drinks, sugar content 19
sugar 16–22
 cutting down 24
 health effects 18–19, 21
 types 16–17
Sugar Puffs, complaints about marketing 29–30
sugar reduction campaign 20
sweeteners 11
Swizzles, complaints about marketing 30

television advertising of junk food 27–8
Tesco, food education programme 35–6
tobacco use, Victorian era 2
trans fat (hydrogenated fat) 15

undernutrition 4
unsaturated fat 15

Victorian era diet 1–2

waste food 2
water consumption 7, 31
websites and advertising of junk food 28, 29–30
whole grains 23

yeast in Victorian diet 1–2

Acknowledgements

The publisher is grateful for permission to reproduce the material in this book. While every care has been taken to trace and acknowledge copyright, the publisher tenders its apology for any accidental infringement or where copyright has proved untraceable. The publisher would be pleased to come to a suitable arrangement in any such case with the rightful owner.

Images

Cover and pages iii, 1, 7, 12, 18, 31, 37: iStock.

Icons on page 15 are from Flaticon and Freepik.

Illustrations

Don Hatcher: page 30. Simon Kneebone: pages 20 & 24. Angelo Madrid: pages 21 & 32.

Additional acknowledgements

Editorial on behalf of Independence Educational Publishers by Cara Acred.

With thanks to the Independence team: Mary Chapman, Sandra Dennis, Christina Hughes, Jackie Staines and Jan Sunderland.

Cara Acred

Cambridge

September 2014